GW01090808

# BUTTOCKS, BOOBS AND BEDPANS

by

Dorothea Desforges

Published by Buttercup Press
South Cave, East Yorkshire, HU15  2JG

©   Dorothea Desforges

First published in Great Britain 2000
Reprinted 2001

All rights reserved

ISBN 0-9539190-0-5

Gem Desk Top Publishing
Welton, East Yorkshire, HU15  1NP

# Contents

# Introduction

'Exploding bodies.' The headline screamed out at me, here I was sitting in a giant jumbo jet as it lumbered along in a long snaking queue of miscellaneous aircraft. All were heading for the one runway still in operation. Because of the dense fog, air traffic control was allowing only one take-off every five minutes. It was going to be a long and tortuous ride and all hopes of catching my connecting flight in New York was fast disappearing in the swirling mists of Chicago's O'Hare airport.

Many passengers were praying - very loudly. Many, like me, were reading anything to hand, including the safety instructions!

The previous evening I had been to a theatre in Chicago. It was one of those plays beloved of the Americans where, in the interval, the audience decide on the ending. Oh, I wish I'd read the 'exploding bodies' article before the performance. I could just imagine the scenario. The cast would ask: "Ok you guys, what do you think? How should it end?" Ideas would flow fast and furious from the audience... "Stab, poison, shoot, heart attack, even a car crash. Then I would call out, "He explodes." The audience and cast would all turn in my direction. "He explodes!! Go on then how does he manage that?"

I would explain, "He is rushed to hospital and explodes in the operating theatre."

Everyone would be curious and I could have gone on to explain that nitrous oxide - which is sometimes used as an anaesthetic in stomach surgery - can get mixed up with intestinal gasses, and these have proved to be highly combustible in countless scientific experiments. If this mixture is ignited by a spark from a surgical implement the result can be what the article referred to as "intra-abdominal fires".

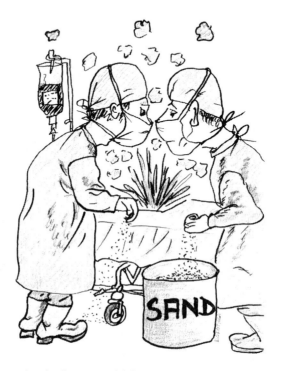

Do you think they would have been impressed?

The article did go on to say that patients aren't exactly exploding all over the place, but it is possible, and can happen to anyone. But don't worry not all explode, some just catch fire! There that makes you feel better doesn't it?

An orthopaedic surgeon once told me he saw a notice above the sink where surgeons scrub up before operating. The heading was - and I'm not making this up - "Emergency procedure; fighting fire on the surgical patient." He said: "It went on to give step-by-step instructions for dealing with different types of fires on a patient and under "large fire on the patient", it gave a very precise instruction'. 'You must care for the patient.' it said. But there was a slight problem," said the surgeon. " It didn't say how."

The writer of the article said he had a vision of a prostrate body laying on the operating table when suddenly, whoosh! he/she explodes. "Call for the fire brigade" yells the surgeon. In minutes, men clad in fluorescent wellies and souwesters barge into casualty, trailing their hose behind them.

"Where's the fire?" yells the chief.

"In the operating theatre."

"Where's that?"

"Through the swing doors, up a flight of stairs, through another door marked 'Fire Exit,' turn right and it's the third door on the left."

But just to digress for a moment. A couple of weeks ago, I was happily sitting in out-patients when the fire alarms sounded. No-one moved. In minutes we had men clad in fluorescent jackets and wellies, charging through the swing doors. The 'fire' was in a small side room, caused by an occupational therapist leaving a small boiler to heat up, and it wasn't smoke, but the steam erupting from the boiling pan.

Karen still hasn't owned up - OOPS!

Anyway back to the operating theatre. Firemen, hoses now primed and ready, burst through the swing doors prepared for action.

"Thank god you've arrived." screams the anaesthetist. "Put out that patient."

He/she is liberally doused and sizzling can clearly be heard. Mission accomplished, the crew stomp out of the theatre, leaving the surgeon to carry on, clad only in his boxer shorts - he'd ripped off his operating gown to smother the offending patient - sorry, I mean fire.

Everything goes smoothly, except when the patient revives, he/she is rather curious as to why their paper knickers are scorched around the edges.

Don't give this matter another thought if you are about to embark on a journey to an operating theatre. I'm sure hospitals will have taken the precaution of installing a sprinkler system above your prostrate body, but as an extra precaution maybe you should arrange for a couple of muscular fire-fighters to be standing by, buckets at the ready.

Puts a whole new meaning to 'throw a bucket of water over him/her, doesn't it?

Oh another thing. Did you know they tape down your wedding ring in the operating theatre? Evidently if there is a mass of static electricity lurking about and if your arm should suddenly flop down, inadvertently touching the metal edge of the operating table, you'll make very pretty lights - and most likely electrocute the surgeon as well as yourself. I was also told it's to stop the ring being filched while you lie there in all your naked glory.

Intestinal gasses can cause other problems too. I remember an article in a newspaper about a Moroccan man who was found dead in bed. The coroner said: "There were no marks on his body, but the autopsy revealed he had large amounts of methane gas in his system. Relatives have confirmed to me that his diet consisted of cabbage and beans, exactly the right combination of foods to produce large quantities of methane."

It appears that he had been repeatedly passing wind and died by gassing himself in his small airtight room.

Absolutely true. You couldn't make that up could you?

Seriously, I'm sure your operation will go just fine and you can rest assured that in the event of an explosion, no matter how many pieces end up on the ceiling, every one of those pieces will, in accordance with modern medical standards receive an injection. But please don't tell my friend Sheila. She is absolutely terrified of hospitals and in particular needles. Sheila said: "They say to me, 'You'll hardly feel a thing,' and then come at me as if they're harpooning a whale."

"Don't worry," I told her, "It's better than sending Dracula on a cold and windy night to your bedside."

"Don't you believe it," she said, "Dracula might come into my room and suck out all my blood, but at least I would then turn into a bat and get to stay out all night, whereas with an injection all I get is a sore bum."

Not like Rita, a vivacious twenty-seven year old who had been in hospital for over six weeks for a painful course of steroids, all injected into places you wouldn't want to know about! But easily the favourite with both doctors and nurses was her posterior. At the end of the course she reckoned she'd been punctured a hundred and thirty-eight times.

One evening we were waiting for visitors to arrive when she called out to me: "Hey, Dorothea, I've just thought of a way I can keep my two kids quiet tonight - she had two girls, aged three and five - I'll just lift up my nightie, show 'em my bum and tell 'em to join up the dots. They'll have a great time."

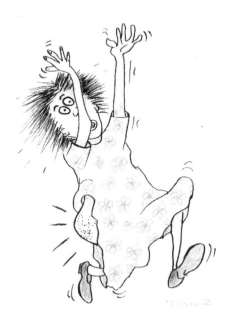

It's now the new millennium and I've just been reading that injections could soon be considered archaic. They've invented something called an 'interject', it's a needle-free injector for liquid drugs.

Whoopee!!

Over the years I have been a 'guest' in several hospitals, where staff and patients have regaled me with anecdotes which kept me amused on many a long night. I heard about a ghost who had a penchant for biting bottom's, a buttercup who was lusted after by a patient in floral pyjamas, fluffy slippers and no teeth, but one of my favourites, told to me by a sister at Hull Royal infirmary, involved a walking corpse. I soon started to keep notes and once staff and patients got to know what I was up to, they bombarded me with tales of the unexpected. Some bizarre, all amusing and many so rude, they would only tell the story if I promised not to divulge the source. I've also heard some wonderful snippets of conversation while sitting obediently in my bed - usually pretending to be asleep! This was a ploy I used when I saw a nurse heading my way with syringe at the ready. Never worked.

I was discussing the amount of needles they stick in various parts of your anatomy, with a patient in the next bed.

"If they stick a needle in my backside, I tell them everything," said Sarah."

"Everything! What do you mean you tell them everything?" I queried.

"Well, I think I do. I'm not sure what happens, but I know yesterday all the staff kept thanking me and they all gave me this knowing smile when they walked by."

Daily I watched desperately ill people admitted to hospital. They seemed to be on their last legs, but a week later were doing cartwheels down the middle of the ward.

Mainly because the medical profession is becoming increasingly adept at keeping the population alive and well, but what we can't possibly even guess at, is when these individuals are 'sorted', what they will do with the rest of their lives.

Roald Dahl told a story of an obstetrician who, by using all his skill, managed to deliver a healthy baby, where perhaps nine out of ten other consultants would have failed. When all was over he asked the mother what she was going to call her baby.

She beamed at the doctor and answered "Adolph."

"That's a nice name Mrs Hitler," said the obstetrician.

Also while perceiving my fellow patients, I found it quite amazing that most of them appeared much less concerned about some feat of surgery about to be performed upon them under anaesthesia, than the fact they couldn't sleep or their meal was cold. But without doubt the one moan which can be heard daily throughout the land is: "Nurse, my bowels wont open."

It's always lovely to see friends and relatives while you're languishing in bed and they invariably arrive bearing a selection of weird and wonderful gifts.

Penny, my son's girlfriend, said she thought I looked a bit green about the gills, so brought me a two-foot high fluffy, green hippo. As the weeks went by he was joined by mice, rabbits, seals, giraffes, pigs, cats and monkeys - all of the cuddly toy variety -

Joanne, an ex-dance band singer, who has a thousand stories to tell of life on the road, visited regularly and always brought something suitable. Once she came in clutching a beautifully wrapped parcel. I opened it eagerly. It contained a box of all-bran - I wont go into details! - I told her I'd been innundated by wonderful anecdotes from the nursing staff, so next time she was laden down with drawing books, paper, pens and pencils. My first 'scribblings' were some of Joanne's stories, concerning her time touring ballrooms in the fifties, with twenty musicians. Many risque, all entertaining and confirmed by my husband, a tenor player and vocalist. All I can say is watch out for 'Bands, Booze and Ballrooms.'

Another regular visitor was my friend Mima, a well known actress and equestrian painter, who once arrived clutching a charcoal drawing of her Shetland pony Tuppence and a small pot containing some newly opened snowdrops, freshly dug from her garden.

Bette went one better, she came one day gingerly carrying something wrapped in strong brown paper. I peered inside. She'd brought me a cactus.

"Well I thought it would last a bit longer than flowers," she said " And you needn't water it."

The weekly visit from Alan always brought an individual rose arranged in its own small vase. Another Alan, this time the playwright Plater, would pop in to keep me up to date with his latest scribblings and always left me giggling. ( Again I'm not going into details! )

I even had a visit from MP John Prescott and his wife Pauline. He strode down the ward, weighed down under the largest pot of yellow chrysanthemums I'd ever seen. They were planted in the garden and continued to grow profusely for several years.

As a newcomer you soon get asked your name by other patients. On one occasion I was greeted by a friendly voice which said: "My names Glo., over there is Doreen, then Mabel and next to 'er Annie. What's your name then?"

"Dorothea."

"What sort of bloody name is that? What do you get called?"

"Dorothea" I told her.

"Not by me you dont."

The following week a dark haired, ebony eyed young man was admitted and placed in the bed directly opposite. I smiled

"What do they call you?" he asked.

"Dorothea."

"Oh, how wonderful, I love that name."

I brightened visibly.

"I call my caravan Dorothea."
Well you must admit its different.

I usually listen to the radio while languishing in my bed, but either the head-sets don't work or you can only get one programme, usually the local station, Radio Humberside, and occasionally the hospital station. They are both a source of rich comedic moments, enough I'm pleased to say, to fill another book all on their own. I listened regularly to Peter Adamson's Soapbox programme on Radio Humberside. One Wednesday the topic seemed to revolve around an article in the newspapers the previous day about a lady who had been found alive in a mortuary after being pronounced dead.

Caller: "I'm glad they're not suing the doctor, when he made a mistake telling everybody the lady was dead. I mean he didn't do it on purpose did he?"

Peter: "No, but I think everybody would like some sort of guarantee, that, that's it"

Caller: "Yes I agree, it is a bit worrying isn't it? I think you should leave your body to medical science. Then they'd know for certain."

There was a short silence.

Peter: "You mean they'd know when they made the first incision?"

Caller: "Something like that yes."

The following day Peter was telling his listeners about the time he was laid up in hospital and there was a man at the far end of the ward, who everyone hated.

"He was constantly on the phone," said Peter, "saying things like, `sell conglomerates` and `what about my gilts?` in a very loud voice so everyone could hear. He made us all think he was rich, so we all hated him." He added, "We couldn't even muster a pound postal order between the lot of us."

Another regular presenter was Ian Hunter and on a request programme he informed his listeners: "I'd like to say a big hello to Daisy Clarke, as she's always going in and out of hospital, ladies and gents."

And later in the week he was told on his phone-in that, "My son-in-laws, brother's an orthopaedic surgeon. He cuts off peoples legs and things."

Two days later a lady came on the phone-in and when the presenter asked how she was, got very enthusiastic and told him she'd been to swimming and keep-fit classes that morning, going on to tell him she had only gone originally because the doctor had given her a prescription for keep-fit classes: "And I liked it so much I kept on going after the prescription ran out."

"Ah so you obviously thought it a good idea then." said the presenter.

"What?"

"The prescription."

"No, not really, it's the keep-fit I like, not the prescription."

"Oh I see," said a baffled presenter.


I worked for many years as a travel agent and a United Airlines stewardess told me about the time she had to ask if there was a doctor on board. "I knew all the passengers expected a Harley Street surgeon to waft through from first class." she said. "Not any more. On this transatlantic flight, the emergency plea for medical aid was answered by a small but perfectly formed figure of a Chinese herbalist, Dr Guo Yao Yu."

"Clutching not a Gladstone bag, but a tub of Tiger Balm, I watched as Dr Yu massaged the exotic contents into the temples and lips of the stricken victim, resulting in a miraculous recovery."

I wonder if the world's airlines will follow suit and will only take-off with a homeopath on board.


Names always intrigue me. A doctor in Hull told me he once worked under a surgeon with the name of Mr Death. "I bet his waiting list was pretty short," I quipped.

"Well, no. He was actually very popular," he said, "No-one realised, as he spelt and pronounced it De'Ath."

When I was in New York I remembered seeing a gynaecological advertisement. The name of the consultant? Dr Ovary.

Also in New York a firm of dentists called, Pullery and Fillery, but nearer to home there is a dentist called D. Kaye, also locally, I saw a wonderful sign outside a dental surgery. It read: 'Patients parking only - Trespassers will be given an appointment.'.

# ACCIDENT & EMERGENCY

My first experience with A&E came after an encounter with a potato. I was foolishly slicing away as it sat snugly in the palm of my hand. I only succeeded in lopping off the end of a finger. The poor thing was hanging by a thread, so my husband bundled me into the car and rushed me to hospital. I tried 'manfully' to be brave - In the new modern world, I expect that would be considered politically incorrect, but womanly doesn't quite have the same ring to it - Anyway there I was bleeding profusely into my Mother-in-law's favourite white blouse, which was wrapped tightly round my hand. I was seen quite quickly, the bleeding stemmed and my wound cleaned. "The doctor will be along in a minute," said the nurse and left me with my throbbing finger. I was wondering if my husband would be allowed to join me in my cubicle, when I heard a voice outside.

"Can you go to cubicle three, there's an elderly patient waiting for stitches."

I thought 'Poor old soul' and wondered what had happened. To my horror a doctor pulled open my curtains and I realised the nurse had meant me. This hurt me far more than any piddling cut. You might say he added insult to injury - I was 47!

I told him I objected to being called elderly.

"Oh, I'm sure she didn't mean anything by it," he said. "In fact, I bet you were a stunner when you were younger."

I told him. "That's what they call digging yourself a hole."

16

It was Sunday lunch time and the emergency department was visibly short on patients, so I told the doctor I would forgive him if he could tell me a funny story about his work.

"I'm not very good on funny," he said.

"Ok, what about macabre, weird or even downright barmy. I'm not particular."

He visibly brightened. "Ah, I can help you there," he said. "In fact only yesterday we had a young man admitted to casualty and he had a really nasty knife wound and was losing copious amounts of blood. One of the nurses checked his wallet and found a card saying he was a Jehovah's Witness, so we knew he couldn't be given a blood transfusion. I went to have a word with the young girl he'd come in with. 'He's not a Jehovah's Witness, she told me. I've no idea where he got the card from'. We rang his parents and they confirmed what his girlfriend had told us, so we went ahead with the transfusion. It turned out that he was an out and out thief and had nicked the wallet while shopping in Hull."

"That's what I want," I told him. "Any more?" He thought for a moment then giggled. "Well we did have one very embarrassed 64 year old admitted with a vibrator stuck up his backpassage."

As I told him. "There's no answer to that."

He suddenly remembered the time another elderly man had been admitted with a broken arm and several cuts on his arms and face. "I knew it was a motoring accident," he said, "so asked him what had happened. "I sneezed." said the patient. I thought he was having me on, or had a head injury I wasn't aware of.

"No, honest," he said, "I suffer from hay fever and as I was driving past a rape field, I started sneezing. One was so violent it made my false teeth fly out and they smashed the windscreen." How did that cause the broken arm?" I asked.

"Oh, I was so bloody shocked by the whole thing I lost control and drove straight into a tree."

The doctor sudenly flashed me an impish grin and asked,

"What do they give a parrot with a headache?"

"I don't know what do they give a parrot with a headache?"
"Parrotcetamol!"

"Heard it," I told him. "You've got to do better than that."

"I know what," he said, "Tell the readers that I'm a poor, over-worked, under-paid doctor who would be neither if I had a pound every time a patient says 'Pardon' when I ask them if their hearing is okay. I wouldn't mind but everyone thinks they are being original. But I did have one lady who grabbed my stethoscope and yelled 'Boo!' into the end. I thought my ear drums had burst. All she did was giggle uncontrollably. But what really annoys me is when I say to the patient 'What brought you here then? and they invariably answer car, ambulance or I walked.'

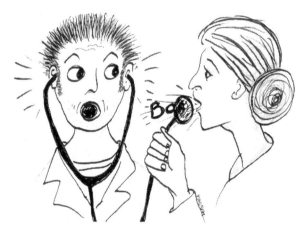

I thanked him and started to walk out when he stopped me: "Another thing about patients," he said, "Over half of them think they'll drop down dead if I ask them to take their vest off."

"Good job you never met my Granddad Hudson then," I replied, "He would never take his cap off. Except once. He'd gone to Boothferry Park to see Hull City with two of his sons. It was pouring down and Granddad took his cap off. "Put your cap on Dad, you'll catch your death of cold." said Norris. "What and ruin my cap?" replied Granddad.

A few years later Grandma persuaded him to buy a new one for my wedding. He never took it off all day, sitting proudly throughout the reception with it perched jauntily on his curly, grey locks.

My doctor friend had one last parting shot. "Did you know," he asked me, "That red ants smell like a fart when they are squashed?"

It was definitely time to depart.

As I was heading through the automatic doors, my friend Claire walked in with her sister Mavis and a small boy in tow with a saucepan stuck on his head.

I stopped to enquire what had happened.

"You would not believe what we've been through. Our Mavis did everything she could to try and dislodge it. This thing only happens in movies. I told her she'd have to bring him to hospital. You wont believe what she did. Only brilloed the bottom of the pan before she would set foot out of the door."

The perfect end to a fun packed day!

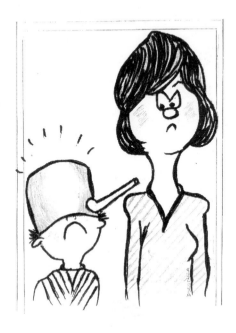

Another time a friend accompanied me when I went to have my plaster casts removed. - I had broken both arms while luxuriating on an island called Bitter End in the Caribbean and just like in the movies, a handsome stranger came to my rescue. It was only Richard Branson - but that's another story - Anyway as I was handing in my appointment card, I noticed a form with the initials B.I.W.D in large letters across the top.

I told Bette and we spent the next twenty minutes trying to work out what it might mean. We eventually gave up and asked a nurse. She gave us a funny smile. "Do you really want to know?" she asked and smiled again. "They stand for 'brought in wrongly dead,' she said.

"How can you be wrongly dead?" asked Bette.

"Don't ask," said the nurse.

"All right I won't if you have a funny story"

She thought for a moment then shook her head. "Sorry, but it's not a bundle of laughs in here." As I turned away I heard her say: "Unless you count last week when a patient was seen to have a black spot on his skull x-ray that the doctor couldn't recognise. He asked for another x-ray and it turned out the spot was a fly on the lens of the camera."

While we were waiting, a twenty something girl was admitted with knife wounds. She was in an absolute fury, screaming to anyone who would listen, how much she hated men, especially Greek ones. "I've been beaten and humiliated and this is the last straw," she yelled, then threatened to do great damage to any Greek male she ever came into contact with again. The nurse was trying to clean the fairly superficial wounds when the male doctor went to check if the injury needed stitching. He was Greek!

Nearby a young man returned to sit near us. "What did the doctor say?" asked his anxious partner. With a totally straight face he said: "Take it easy, be waited on hand and foot and have sex twice a day."

Bette looked excitedly at me. "Whatever he's got, I want." she said.

I was relating the 'pan' story to Bette and she told me it reminded her of the time the family had gone on holiday to Scotland. She said, "I had to rush my four year old to hospital. He'd pushed a pea up each nostril, I sat with the doctor while he tried to remove them. He eventually managed to get them out and he asked my son why he'd put the peas up his nose. I was flabbergasted when he told the young doctor, "Because they kept falling out of my ears."

# AMBULANCE DRIVERS

My father worked in the ambulance brigade for many years, long before paramedics were even thought about. He started off as a driver and ended his career as Station Officer.

Dad told me: "When people ring up they are usually in an agitated state and come out with the most extraordinary remarks. I remember asking a patient what was wrong and he told me. 'Ooh, it's bad guv., I can't breathe, in fact I haven't been able to for years.' Another time a patient told my mate, 'I'm glad you came so quick. I'm under the doc. and I can't breathe."

He laughed. "One lady was advised that an ambulance was on its way, so she told the telephonist. 'Well I hope you send a driver with the ambulance 'cos my husband is useless."

"We'd gone to one house on Anlaby Road to pick up a lady who'd collapsed. A young man rushed up to meet me as I got out of the ambulance and told me: 'If my mother goes in that ambulance without me I'll kill her." But he said his favourite was when an elderly lady explained: "My husband is dead so he'll not be able to bring me in."

During one drive to the hospital he said he was making conversation with an elderly lady who had a suspected broken femur. Dad said: "I asked her when her birthday was, she told me June 15th. What year? I asked her and she looked at me as if I was mad and replied 'Every year of course."

There had been a very nasty incident in the city centre and several ambulances were called for. One man had been severely beaten up and was laid in a pool of blood on the pavement. The ambulance men placed his crumpled body on a stretcher and rushed him to hospital. As they wheeled the man into casualty a doctor asked them. "Did you check his pulse?" "Yes," replied an ambulance man, "but he was obviously dead." The doctor persevered. "Did you check his breathing?" he asked. At this an exasperated driver told him. "It was a bit difficult with his head smashed in."

At that moment another patient was being rushed through to casualty. He was asked if he had been "injured in the fracas." "No," replied the man, "I was hurt in the small of my back."

Tony Richards was another well known character in the service.

"No matter how long you can be attending a patient," he said, "they never remember you, even if you meet them a few weeks later, it always surprised me, but there was one exception. It was my first day as an ambulance man and we had been called to a young boy who'd been in a road accident. His leg was in a real state and we were convinced it couldn't be saved. We splinted and bandaged him, all the while calming his mum and telling her he'd be playing football in weeks. Four or five YEARS later, I was walking through the fracture clinic when a lady approached me. "You don't remember me do you?" she asked. At first I didn't but when she reminded me of the accident the penny dropped. She told me 'I'll never forgot you, you cheered me up so much, when I was so worried. That really chuffed me," said Tony, "As it was the first day on a completely different career move."

He carried on with his reminiscences: "Dogs were often a problem when we were attending emergencies and my mate Dave was terrified of them. We'd been called out late one evening and I was driving - we took it in turns - As he rang the bell, dogs immediately started growling and barking from behind the door.

He shouted through the letter-box for the owners to call the dogs away. The lady inside just kept telling him there wasn't a problem and would he please 'just get inside.' But Dave insisted she got rid of the dogs first. 'It's all right now,' shouted the lady and Dave opened the door and there she stood with two small dogs tucked under each arm. As soon as they saw Dave they started barking again, then one promptly turned and bit his mistress on her breast, so we ended up taking her to hospital for a tetanus jab."

"A few weeks later we'd been called to a house and when I went upstairs a young girl of fourteen was about to give birth. No-one in the family knew a thing about it. A doctor was with her and asked if we would wait downstairs ready to take her to hospital. Dave decided to stay in the cab as a very large dog could be seen prowling around inside. I sat on a settee and it positioned itself in front of me, The thing had a head the size of a lion's. 'Don't worry, ' said a male sitting nearby, 'it's soft as a brush.' Oh yes, where have I heard that before! It was eyeing me up as if I was a tasty dinner but I still persuaded Dave to come inside for a cup of tea. As soon as he entered the room it started growling and baring it's teeth. Dave didn't wait to see if he was on the menu."

"I think one thing that really irritated all of us was the amount of dog muck we stepped in while attending emergencies. It would get on the floor, on the pedals, in fact everywhere, the smell was foul. And strange, but if you asked, it couldn't possibly be their dog. 'Mine never does it outside,' or 'we always scoop it up.' We got so fed up we decided to write to the letters page of the local newspaper. We thought we'd be inundated with protests or letters defending us, but we only got one letter and that was from an irate reader who asked 'Who do these ambulancemen think they are, they ought to go to East park sometime and see the mess the ducks make."

"I remember being called out to an old lady who'd fallen. When we arrived she was laid out on the mat in the front room, a man in his thirties stood nearby. "Where did she fall, was it here?' we asked.'Oh, no,' the young man answered, 'I put her here.' We persevered. 'Where then, in the hall?' 'Oh no, it was round the corner in the next road. I had to carry her back.' He obviously thought he's done the proper thing. I didn't say anything while we were attending to the badly shaken patient, who we diagnosed as having a broken femur, but after we'd put on the splints and placed her on a stretcher I couldn't help telling the young man how dangerous it was to move anyone who was obviously injured. 'You could have killed her' I told him. 'Sorry guv.' he said, 'I thought I was helping.'

"Three weeks later, at two in the morning, we'd been called out to a traffic accident. It was pouring down and we could just see a figure huddled in the middle of the road. I bent over him about to ask some questions when a hand landed on my shoulder and a voice behind me said, 'I didn't touch him guv. I remembered what you said, so I never touched him."

"We had some real laughs," confessed Tony, "One time we radioed in to the control room and told the boss we had a problem. Our ambulance would only work in one gear, - reverse. 'Where are you?" he asked, we told him at the Hull Royal, which was about a mile away. Even though it was three am in the morning he said "Stay where you are I'll try to get the workshop out." About twenty minutes later we drove backwards into the station. The boss came out to meet us. 'Is it all right now lads?' No, we told him, we had to drive all the way back in reverse. He was duly impressed, pleased he didn't have to call out the engineers and we could have another ambulance. He then told us to go into the control room and file a report. I started writing and asked what I should say. 'Just what you've told me. You can only get reverse.' he said. I wrote it down as requested then asked him for the date. April the first, he replied, then the penny dropped!"

"In the spring we'd been called to a wedding party. We pushed our way through the crowds of guests to a chair where a small elderly man was sitting. "His legs are killing him," said a broad, burly man. "What's wrong pops?" I asked, but the man beside him kept repeating 'It's his legs, they're killing him.' Let him tell us mate, and asked the old man again what was troubling him. 'They should never have called you', he said,'I told them not to.'

"Look we want you to take him to hospital,' said an even larger fellah. We told them, if he doesn't want to go, we can't make him. 'You're taking him', they said and were becoming rather threatening, but the man insisted he was not being taken anywhere. As I was telling them again that we couldn't make him go, all Hell let loose and these two brothers started scrapping, then everybody joined in, even the women. They were hurling bottles at each other, it was absolute mayhem, so we scurried back to the ambulance without the man and called the police to sort it."

"We'd been called out to an emergency at the Station Hotel, as a man had been dancing with another woman and his girl-friend had fiercely objected by pushing a glass into his face. We were helping him into the ambulance when she re-appeared. The man was screaming, 'I don't want her in here, get her off.' We tried to persuade her to get off but she was one angry lady. My mate had to physically pull her out from the ambulance and as he was pulling up the steps she kicked out at him, right between the legs. He doubled up like a concertina and I had to put him in the back as well. I arrived at the hospital and as soon as the patient stepped down from the ambulance this girl was waiting in the casualty entrance and started setting about him again. She'd evidently rushed round the corner from the hotel, jumped in a taxi and had got there ahead of us."

"One story might make you laugh," said Tony. "I'd been asked to take a mental patient to Brandesburton Hospital by car. He was built like a house-side so I decided that if he was at the back I couldn't keep an eye on him, so opted for him to sit in the front with me. During the journey he kept offering me sweets from a packet. I kept saying no, but he was getting rather aggressive at my refusals, so decided I'd better take a sweet when it was offered. He never touched them himself. When we arrived at the hospital I took him through to the relevant ward and he immediately rushed up to a nurse shouting, 'That driver pinched all my sweets."

"They say an ambulance man lifts every patient, on average, eight times before he gets settled into a hospital bed." said Tony. "No wonder they all have back problems, including me." He went on to tell me about the time they were called out to a rugby match. "We were led to the back of the stands, up some stairs, along a corridor, up some more steps, through the bath and shower area, along a narrow, dark corridor and into a dark, poky room. Lying on a bench was the biggest guy I've ever seen in my life. He must have been six foot three and, about twenty stone - by the way I'm five foot eight and ten stone wet through. We were told he had a suspected back injury. I asked them where it happened. 'On the pitch' said a small diminutive man, with spectacles. So I asked him why the hell didn't he leave him on the pitch, we have to get him back down again now. It took four of us to manoeuvre man mountain back along those stairs and passages."

# CALL OUT

A doctor was discussing the strange reasons patients ask for a night visit. "I vividly remember one particular night." he said, "mainly because it was bitterly cold, bucketing down with rain and I'd already had more than my fair share of time wasters."

"It had started at midnight when a lady rang to tell me, 'When I close my mouth, I can't breathe out.' Can you believe that? I'd just got to sleep when the phone rang again. It was 2.00am and a hysterical woman insisted I went to see her. When I arrived, she told me she'd had dreamt she had cancer and wanted a cervical smear immediately."

"Come 3.30am and an eighteen stone construction worker rang for 'something to ease the pain of his cold sore!' I was not a happy GP."

"At 7.15 I'd just got up as I had to be at the surgery at 8.30am. I was in the shower when I heard the flaming phone again. The wife answered it and came to tell me it was a patient who needed a repeat prescription, but I had to sanction the medication."

"Tell her she has to come to the surgery, as I have to see her." The message was passed on. She told my wife I had to visit her."

"Ask her why?"

"My wife's face was a picture when she related the reply to me. 'She says, she's fine but her hairs a mess."

"But it didn't end there. Five minutes before leaving home the phone went again. "I've just remembered I need you to sign my passport application. Can you come round?"

Gordon, a well respected G.P was called out to a local disco. "I understand it had the reputation of being the hottest spot in town," said Gordon.

"When I arrived the noise was deafening and no-one knew about the emergency call so I made my way to the back and pulled aside a heavy velvet curtain. In the gloom I could make out three or four figures all swigging from bottles and a prostrate figure on the floor. I knelt beside him, but because of the noise I couldn't hear anything, nor could I feel a pulse. I got within inches of his face and screamed 'Are you dead?' It worked, the 'corpse' shook his head, stood up, muttered, 'bloody 'ell, what happened?' One of the beer drinkers, muttered, 'serves you bloody right, you kissed the mike and the bloody thing was live.' With that he leapt up and went back on stage. I packed up my bag and found the only way back was across the stage. I was greeted with loud cheering, whistles and applause. My head was banging when I eventually made it through the sweaty, shouting throng. Thank goodness I was born sixty years ago."

A local G.P told me about the time a pensioner contacted him.
"It was 2.00am, she said it was an emergency and she sounded quite perturbed. When I arrived she was sat in a high backed chair, drinking a cup of tea. She seemed fine. I asked what the problem was."
"I've got wax in my left ear and it needs syringing."
Asked why she hadn't waited and made an appointment at the surgery, she answered.
"Why should I? I've gone deaf in that ear, so I consider that an emergency."
"I'd just settled down when I was called out again. An agitated female asked 'Can you come and see my husband he's in

29

real pain.' When I arrived at the address I just knocked and walked in. I was faced with a man in his thirties, wearing only a Manchester United shirt. He gave me a strange look, stuck his bum in the air and said: 'Can you look at my piles Doc.? They're giving me jip tonight."

"An hour later I was heading to a small holding on the edge of town. A rather upset lady had told me. ' I think Tommy has broken his leg doctor."

I was met at the door by an anxious young woman. 'He's in the kitchen.' I followed her into a large room, with the brown Aga in the corner exuding a comforting warmth. She pointed to a large cushion. "There's Tommy.' she said."

"It's a dog."

"Of course it is. Just have a look and see what you think."

"But I'm a doctor. Why didn't you call a vet?"

"Oh, I didn't like bothering him."

"It must be something about animals," he said, because a week later, about 4.30am, the phone jangled me into consciousness. I was already having 'one of those nights' so this time I made doubly sure what I was letting myself in for. A good job I did. This time would you believe, they were calling me out because the cat had got stuck in the cat flap."

It was eight o'clock in the evening and Dr G... had been called out to a lady who'd been vomiting all day.

"I was alarmed at the dark brown mass she'd been bringing up and thought she could be haemorrhaging, so called an ambulance."

"At the Hull Royal Infirmary, questions were asked and the 'sick' examined. They were puzzled. It definitely wasn't blood. She was asked what she had for tea the previous day. 'Scrambled egg,' came the reply. "Nothing else?" No,' the patient replied then suddenly looked very sheepish. "Ooohh, I remember now. I bought a packet of yoghurt covered raisins in Marks & Spencers and ate the lot before I got back to my car."

Problem solved.

"Do you mind getting called out at night?" I asked.

"No, not really, we take it in turns and you arrange your life to suit. We're only the same as many others who work nights." He laughed. "Which reminds me, last week I had to call out a plumber at midnight. He was about an hour fixing the leak and I asked how much? When he told me, I nearly went into shock, that's more than twice I get for night calls I told him. 'I can believe it, he said, that's why I gave up general practice."

# CHIROPODY

Jayne Partridge is a chiropodist in a local store. She said many clients use their time on the couch to divulge their innermost secrets. "They consider me a sort of closet psychologist and often tell me the most amazing things. I had a lady in yesterday who'd just returned from a cruise to the Canary Islands. On the second day she inadvertently flushed her false teeth down the loo." Jayne started to giggle. "She told me the captain had told her he would flush out the bilge tank to see if he could find them. My client said she didn't fancy that, so continued toothless for the rest of the voyage."

"I do get a lot of elderly patients," confessed Jayne, "and they sometimes come up with the most outrageous comments. Yesterday I was chatting to Mrs Watson and she asked me if I'd seen the hospital programme the previous night. I told her I hadn't. 'Oh, it was really good,' she told me, 'they showed a hernia operation, the one my husband's having done next week. It looks a bit nasty to me Jayne. I thought knee hole surgery was uncomplicated.' I had to explain that I think she meant keyhole surgery."

Helen was a chiropodist who visited patients in their homes. "I had one lady who was a tiny little thing. About four foot ten or so. She would sit on a chair dangling her legs like a child in a high chair, just managing to rest them on a special pink satin, heart shaped cushion. Her feet were delicate and always beautifully manicured. Whenever anyone came to visit they always had to let her try their shoes on, male or female, then would parade around exclaiming: "Look what big feet you've got."

On every visit I had to tell her how perfect her feet were."

Patricia was another who only did home visits. "I was asked to visit an elderly lady in a small terraced house. I knocked at the door and was met by the daughter and a large ginger tom."

"Do you mind cats?" she asked.

"No, not at all I told her and followed her into the house and was immediately overpowered by the stench of urine, very stale urine"

"I set up my stool and arranged the equipment. The lady put her foot on the stool then suddenly called to her daughter. "Let the others in now."

"The girl went to a door which led to a small kitchen, as it was opened a horde of cats rushed forward."

"They climbed in my bag which was filled with sanitised equipment, jumped onto my knees, one even leapt onto my shoulders. There were fourteen of them, all with free range of the house. I finished in double quick time," said Patricia, "and decided I wouldn't accept any other requests to visit. But I needn't have worried, they never rang again for another appointment."

Patricia also told me about a regular client who she visited every three months just to trim her nails and sort out a maverick corn now and again.

"Her feet were unbelievably soft and smooth. I once asked her how she kept them in such wonderful condition. Her reply surprised me to say the least. She told me she massaged them every day with double cream."

"But that had nothing on Albert. I knew he'd been in hospital so thought I'd pop round and see how he was. He was just about to give his feet a good old soak. I told him to carry on.

He crumbled a cube of bath salts into an orange washing-up-bowl, then slowly lowered his size tens into the steaming water. His eyes were tight shut and he had a look of complete contentment on his face. He insisted I stay and asked me to make a drink for him. He paddled his feet around, slopping water onto the carpet while we chatted and he drank his tea. He then lifted his feet out, towelled them down and started to massage them with a disgusting green, jelly-like substance. It smelt as revolting as it looked. I asked him what it was but he just tapped the side of his nose, winked and said, 'That's for me to know and you to find out. All I want you to do is trim my nails and cut out my corns, you can leave the important jobs to me'"

"I didn't argue and I still haven't a clue what he was putting on his feet"

# CONSULTANTS

Trevour, a young medical student, who had just had a run-in with a rheumatologist, spoke with feeling when he was telling me about consultants. "I only understood half of what he was talking about." He shook his head. "I wouldn't be surprised if half of the consultants in the country are first taken into theatre for a meaningless jargon implant before they're let loose on medical students."

I know what he means. I was a patient for seven months in ward seventy of The Hull Royal Infirmary, so got to know many staff intimately - in the nicest possible way of course!- This was the time of the dreaded Matron and when consultant's made their rounds they were followed by a retinue of the great and good.

My consultant was Dr. Goode, a tall, gentle man, not a bit like one of his compatriots, who shall be nameless, but you could feel the pomposity as he strode through the ward like a drill sergeant. When he stopped by a bed, the whole party would jump to attention as if they were soldiers on parade.

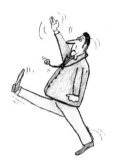

Like all the others, Dr Goode also did his rounds followed by his retinue. First in line would be his registrar, behind him a house surgeon and a house doctor followed by sister, then a senior staff nurse, who was usually in charge of a tray of instruments. I usually got tapped, occasionally tickled and all limbs were invariably stretched and manipulated. Dr Goode would hold meaningful conversations with his registrar and the sister. If he needed to explain in detail, large sheets of paper would be produced for him to draw diagrams. He told everyone about the problem, except the patient, which of course was normal in those days. It took nearly three months for him to relax and stand beside my bed and hold significant discussions with me.

Although one day he had anything but an interchange of ideas with the lady in the bed next to me. He checked through her notes and raised an x-ray to look at it more closely, then turning to her commented: "Mmm, very unusual for a lady. It's your cartilage isn't it?"

"Naw, not me doc." she replied, "I'm in wiv me leg."

The young houseman gave a discernible giggle, but everyone else ignored this little gem, so he suddenly found something interesting in the notes he was carrying. They huddled at the end of the bed. Sister made some notes and as the retinue walked towards the next patient, Sister told her. "We're going to arrange a physiotherapist to see you tomorrow."

"I'm not going to 'ave me leg off am I?"

"No, not today anyway."quipped Sister and quickly rejoined Dr Goode's assemblage.

He had even less joy with the next patient, who was having breathing problems, caused by obesity. Again the team handed him the patients notes and after checking them mentioned to his registrar: "It doesn't look as though Mrs Peel has been weighed."

"Tell him I 'aven't," she shouted. "I told the nurse I don't get weighed if I've got constipation.

36

She was told it was important they knew her weight.

"You bloody doctors are all the same." she said. "Lose weight, lose weight, you say, I'm only seventeen stone. It's in me genes, I can't do nuthin' about it. I knew somebody who dropped dead with a heart attack 'cos 'e exercised"

"How long is it since you were weighed?" asked Sister.

"I like being fat, if you're not, in later life you bloody sag don't you? I don't give a sod. I hate me sister-in-law, she's always telling me about bloody Americans and cholesterol, she says things like, if you don't 'ave salt, you'll snuff it."

Dr Goode started to look rather uncomfortable but asked:

"Is your sister-in-law American?"

"No she's bloody English. English! and behaving like that. Do you know what she brought me back from America?"
The whole retinue waited for the answer, as well as half the ward. She didn't let us down.

"She only brought me a bloody book on American diets. It was rubbish. What's the matter with English stuff, that's what I'd like to know. She's only bragging 'cos she's a size 14. I think she looks like an escapee from Belsen."

I never did see her get weighed.

Another consultant was incredibly good looking, and when this moustachioed smoothie walked through the doors, he radiated confidence like a lighthouse in the thick of a storm. He always wore a rose in his buttonhole and the tip of a spotted handkerchief, folded into a triangle, peeping out of his breast pocket. He exuded an easy authority. Of course all the nurses were madly in love with him, but like all the others, he still paraded with his 'troops'.

One Tuesday afternoon, the team were heading for a red-haired lady who was looking decidedly cross.

"How are you feeling Mrs Betts?"

"I thought you said I was here for a rest."

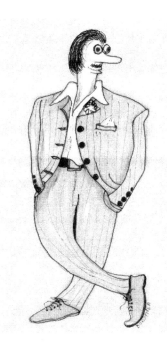

"That's right." said the consultant. "It's very important you get plenty of rest."

"Rest! Some rest I'm getting. I'm never left alone. I've been prodded and poked 'till I'm fed up with it. I just start nodding off and they want to do something else to me. You call that rest!"

In his usual way, he appeased the patient but the staff were not so lucky. He would suddenly fire off a question to one of the retinue and stare fixedly while they struggled for coherence. I watched fascinated as one day a young houseman, paused, swallowed hard then blurted out the answer. The consultant nodded and smiled, they were all obviously in complete awe of the man, you felt they wouldn't be surprised if he'd suddenly yelled 'abra cadabra' and produced a pair of doves from up his sleeve, and he had a wicked sense of humour. One day while on his rounds, they all stopped at the end of a bed, containing Maisie, a sprightly 87 year old, who appeared asleep. "Good morning Mrs Shaw. Are you awake?" Maisie opened her eyes: "Oh, yes, I was just resting my eyes, doctor."

"Thank goodness for that," replied the consultant. "I get worried when people of your age don't move."

A small, dapper, consultant was so pale and thin, you couldn't believe he was giving US advice on how to improve our health. A curtain was slightly ajar one day and I watched as he tapped a patients breasts with a long, slender finger, as if he was checking for ripe melons at the supermarket. Most peculiar.

Alice, an auxiliary nurse summed him up beautifully: "He could take somebody's place in the mortuary and I don't think anybody would notice," she said.

Many of the patients were suffering from leg ulcers and a consultant was telling Mrs Jackson that he was changing her treatment.

The lady in the next bed called out. "Don't you let 'em do it. They put that stuff on me. It set like a broken arm. You tell 'er what 'appens then.. You 'ave to chop it off wiv an 'ammer dont you?"

Phil Hammond, a doctor who writes a regular column in the Daily Express was commenting on what clothes a doctor wore. As he so succinctly put it, "If you'd seen the same G.P for years, you wouldn't care if he was naked as long as he hands over some pills and a sicknote."

He went on to say that in hospitals patients are more concerned with whether they're going to die or when lunch is coming.

"Some consultants however insist their juniors are smartly turned out." He says he knows of one surgeon, "who sends all his male junior doctors off the wards if they are not wearing a silk tie (with Windsor knot ) and brogues."

This has all been very sexist, hasn't it? But twenty years ago, I never met one female consultant. Now they are no longer a rarity, but I'm afraid the stories about them are, let's hope I have a few for my next publication.

While waiting to go into X-ray I heard a nurse ask a patient which consultant she was waiting to see.

"No idea," she replied

"What is he a specialist in?"

"Not sure. Something to do with illnesses."

# DISTRICT NURSES

District nurses are all things to all men - and women - One used to visit me on a daily basis and I got to know her well. Her area was wide and her patients varied. After taking copious amounts of blood from me she had to call on an octogenarian who lived happily on her own, but who had recently fallen and had refused to go into hospital preferring the friendly and helpful advice the district nurse could give her.

Christine told me: "I'd been given a thermometer to test the temperature of water before any patients plunged in. I was helping an elderly lady to bathe and as she was getting ready to climb in, I stopped her, explaining that I had to test her water first."

'Oh,' said Ethyl, shall I pee in the bucket at the side of the bath then?"

Chris. also told me she used to visit a gentleman, at the beginning of each month who never failed to make her laugh."

"Why, did he tell jokes?"

"Oh no," chuckled Christine, it was the way he changed subjects. I could never keep up with him."

I asked if she could give a for instance. She thought for a moment, then laughed.

" I remember him telling me about his wife Sheila, who was once engaged to an Australian sheep farmer, 'but I'm pleased to say,' he said, 'she abandoned him for me.' and without pausing for breath told me he thought his wife was the most wonderful woman in all the world. 'She plays the flute you know and she absolutely hates onions."

Now that's changing subjects!

Janice had to pay a weekly visit to an old gentleman. "Before I opened the door, I knew I would be greeted by the smell of rancid urine. Mainly from the cats. It permeated walls, carpets and furniture. The old man always wore a disintegrating, grey aertex vest. His trousers were indistinguishable flimsy, material, and because he wore no underpants, his 'paraphernalia' was silhouetted quite clearly underneath. I've never seen balls so huge in all my fifteen years of nursing. I always wondered if he'd stuck a couple of oranges and a banana down there just to impress me!

"While in the house, I would try not breathe through my nose, but I never succeeded, just one deep breath and wow!!"

Michael Everard, a Charge Nurse in a surgical ward, said he had a patient who had been discharged from hospital after a successful hip replacement. A district nurse used to visit him every three or four days to change his elasticised stockings. After six weeks the stockings could be discarded for good.

"Are you pleased?" asked the nurse.

"I'll say," answered William.

"And nothing else worrying you?"

"Well there is one thing."

"Oh, what's that?"

"Just a little thing," said William, "But is it all right for me to take my plastic name bracelet off now?"

One nurse told me about a house where the elderly lady was scrupulously clean but she never seemed to touch her window sills. "They were littered with the corpse's of every insect imaginable, going back years! Oooh, and there was Mrs Chapman. I suppose you could say she was a lady of indeterminate years. She was always wearing a shortie, blue checked night-gown, with large puffy sleeves. She was permanently washing and cutting vegetables, especially cucumber, which was always rancid. She would squeeze it and eject the froth into a chipped saucer, then wipe it through her dyed, jet-black hair, which was arranged like skeins of wool along her scalp. 'It's good for it.' she would tell me and offer to wipe some through my fair locks, but I always managed some excuse to escape her clutches."

Sounds like a near thing to me.

"Oh, and the pensioner who had to have regular blood tests. She was always wearing her nightie and curlers. Long pendulous breasts could be seen hanging in abject surrender just skimming the top of her navy blue bloomers. She said she didn't like to get dressed until I'd been. It might seem a bit odd but she was a real sparky lady. A real character."

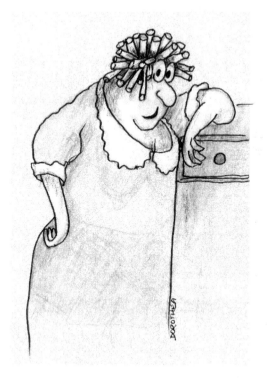

# DOMESTICS

Domestics seem to fall into two camps. The never ending complainers, or the forever chatty, cheerful types.

Beryl was a chatty one. She kept many a mournful patient amused, always ready with a quip to lighten the clouds, but one morning the usually ebullient Beryl came striding into the ward shouting, "Boring, boring, boring, you're all bloody boring."

Everyone looked astounded. She stood surveying the now fully observant ward.

"There, that got your attention didn't it. Usually only two or three bother to say hello, so tomorrow when I say good morning, I want a reply from every one of you miserable lot. Okay?"

Everyone nodded and smiled. Next morning good as their word, Beryl was greeted with a rousing welcome.

A young trainee had left a menu on each bedside table for us to choose the following days meals. I heard Molly ask: "What does sauté mean?"

"Fried." snapped Imogen in the next bed.

"Why doesn't it say fried then?" asked Molly.

"Don't ask me, I'm only telling you."

Suddenly a voice from the end of the ward butted in. "Do like me. Don't put nowt down. I can never make 'ead nor tail of 'em. I live on sandwiches. I'd do that. Just 'ave sandwiches. You can't go wrong then."

"I'm not having sandwiches. I'll have those sauté things They sound real posh."

The voice came from the end of the ward. "You can't tell nobody nothing!"

"You mind your business. I might be common like you but I can pretend I'm posh."

I thought this would be pistols at dawn at the very least but not a word from the sandwich lady.


The domestics were making their daily tea round. Sheila in the next bed asked for black coffee with no sugar.

"Would you like a drop of milk in your black coffee?" asked Carol

The following day I was first on her round.

"Would you like tea or coffee Dorothea?"

"Tea please, milk but no sugar."

"No milk?"

"No, I'd like milk."

"Right. No sugar. Oh dear, I haven't put the tea on the trolley. Are you sure you wouldn't like coffee?"

"All right I'll have coffee. Milk and one sugar."

"Right. Coffee it is. Oh dear, I've forgotten to put milk on the trolley as well, will you have it black?"


Noon, heralded lunch. I watched as they took a plate to Audrey.

She looked at it and asked: "Don't I get vegetables with my chicken pie?"

"Did you ask for vegetables?"

"No, I thought it would be automatic."

"Why should it be automatic?"

"Don't you always have vegetables with your lunch?"

"What with bloody baked beans on toast?"

45

Next morning, while reading my newspaper, I was aware of two cleaners embroiled in an earnest conversation at the end of my bed.

"Didn't you bring your own scrubber?" asked the one with blonde, frizzy hair.

"Well I was going to ..." replied the plump one with the high, arched eyebrows.

"Not to worry, I'll do it without. Is it your turn to strip today?"

"Yes, but I need you to put the polish on."

"Yeah, okay, I like doing that, but I need to have a good going over, it's Tuesday since I had a good one."

"Good. Do that then and we can dry off."

Jackie Collins, eat your heart out.


The tea round was wending it's way to us. "Tea or coffee?"

"I'll have coffee," said Brenda, "But I don't want yours. I've brought my own."

"That's okay," replied the young girl and came to collect the jar. "Ooh, it's Maxwell House. That's the same as we use."

"Well you might say that, but it tastes different."

The girl reached down and produced the jar she normally used to dispense coffee. It was indeed identical.

"I don't care what you say, and it might look the same, but it tastes nothing like my own."

For the next two weeks the patient always insisted they use the contents of her coffee jar.

# ELDERLY

**M**any of the stories I heard were about elderly patients, and during my many visits to hospital I met some pretty weird and wonderful characters of my own. Some oldies can be cantankerous and bloody minded, but many were charming and amusing. I never failed to be impressed by their indomitable spirit.

A Staff nurse told me that the older female patients do not like male nurses: "But the males patients are not so reticent," said Carol, "In sixteen years of nursing only one male has refused to let me touch him. He used to sit on his bed and visibly cower whenever a female nurse approached him, but he was only in for three days so it wasn't much of a problem. Females on the whole

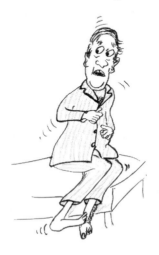

can be quite shy. I remember one lady who was rushed in as an emergency and obviously didn't have her own nightie, so she was given a hospital gown which opened at the back. She was horrified and insisted we took a commode every time she wanted the loo. 'I'm not having everybody looking at my bottom,' she told us. Even my husband can't do that.' "Well she was seventy-nine," said Carol.

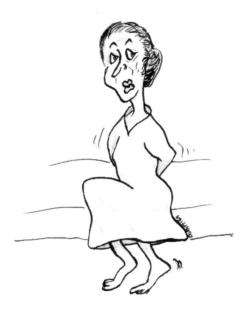

In the Hull Royal Infirmary, Fiona, an auxiliary nurse, would daily have a tale to tell about their senior patients. I'm saying nothing as I now belong to the illustrious ranks of the 'golden oldies!'

Alice was a frail old lady who had been in the hospital for nearly three weeks, during that time Fiona among others, had pandered to her every whim - even to picking out a tissue from a box which was just in front of her and putting it in her hand. On the morning she was due to be discharged Fiona became worried as she could do so little for herself.

She approached Alice and asked if she had any help at home. She said no she was on her own.

"How will you manage?"

"Manage? Why ever shouldn't I manage?" snapped Alice.

"Well it's just that we have to do just about everything for you."

Alice looked pityingly at Fiona. "If you're stupid enough to do it, I'm certainly not stupid enough to refuse."

Fiona said she was so astounded at her reply she just burst out laughing.

On my first day at Castle Hill Hospital I saw Janet rushing over to patient who was walking around her bed.

"What are you doing Amelia? You know you've been told not to walk."

"You said I could sit in my chair."

"You're not sitting, you're walking!"

"Yes, but I'm only walking to my chair."

"But the chair is beside your bed. You're standing on the side without a chair."

"But it's on the wrong side."

"How can it be on the wrong side Amelia? It's a single bed. There isn't a right or wrong side."

"Yes, but I sleep in a double bed at home, so I'm only used to getting out on the left."

Janet moved the chair for her.

Clare Johnston was talking to Mr Gold, a frail, gentle man, who spoke very little. She was chatting to him and asked what sort of things he liked doing. He got very enthusiastic about having a flutter on the "gee-gees"

"Why do you back horses?" asked Clare.

The reply was instant and to the point. "`Cos they don't bloody race giraffes."

A nurse in Castle Hill Hospital said she'd been asked to put a catheter in a 94 year old man. "I went to the bed, pulled back the sheets, looked down and told him, 'Your willy's gone.' He laughed and told me: 'Lady when you get to 94 everything just shrivels up. You know what they say don't you?'

"About what? I asked."

"If you don't use it, you lose it. You're lucky you're a bloody woman."

"I am, why do you say that? I asked him."

"Because when you get to my age and want to go to the loo, you can't get hold of the blasted thing. You ladies don't have that problem."

Mildred was being prepared for an operation and the doctor was checking some details with her. I heard him ask: "Do you wear dentures?"

Mildred nodded her head and said: "Sometimes I have to, but only when I'm reading."

There was a time when nurses were always on the same shifts. If they were on nights, they did it because that was their choice. It was comforting to see the same faces regularly. But today, everyone is expected to work a rotating system. Hated by most nurses and all patients. Having a sign at the end of your bed which pronounces 'named nurse' is supposed to give the patient confidence, except it could be on the seven days off shift, so your "named" nurse will never be seen during your incarceration.

In one hospital my named nurse was shown as Amanda. Three days later she left on maternity leave, ten days after that I was discharged. Amanda's name was still on seven of the ten beds on view. Well she was coming back in four months.

My longest encounter with hospitals was in the eighties when you still had matrons and ward sisters and the same faces were there to comfort you daily.

I particularly enjoyed nights, when they had a little more time to chat. I made friends with many, including Minden who had worked in many environments but was now on permanent nights and was brimming with anecdotes.

She recalled the time she was working in a geriatric ward.

"There were several completely batty old dears who kept everyone awake at night with their antics, so often we would wheel them into a small room nearby and leave them to entertain themselves."

"One evening we were absolutely chokka and were juggling beds around and for a short time had to leave a patient in the corridor. She'd just got to sleep when two ambulancemen came for a quick cup of tea and a natter with Sister. She was on the phone and couldn't chat to them at that moment. The boys saw `the body` and thinking they would be doing sister a favour, decided to wheel it to the mortuary. I just happened to look out into the corridor and realised what they were doing. I walked briskly down the ward - it was instant death if you broke into a trot, let alone run! - Anyway before I had time to even yell, the old biddy sat bolt upright and demanded, `Where the bloody `ell are you taking me now?`

"You should have seen them," she said. "They literally screamed in terror, waking up everybody! It was another two hours before we got the ward all settled down again."

"They had some funny ideas in those days," said Minden. "I remember once the hierarchy decided that to keep some of our patients quiet, we should try letting them suck dummies."

"Dummies! You are joking," I said. "You mean the types given to screaming babies?"

"The same," said Minden. "They thought they'd try it with the elderly patients late at night. They came in a variety of colours. We were issued with pink, yellow and orange for the ladies and blue, purple and grey for the gents."

"It worked then."

"Oh yes. In fact all the nursing staff thought it worked a

treat - I suppose I should say a teat - You should have seen them sitting there happily sucking away."

"It wouldn't do much for their dignity would it?" I ventured.

"I suppose not," said Minden, "but they didn't give a damn and were quite content and happy and that's the important thing isn't it?"

I couldn't argue with that.

The following afternoon I watched Sadie, an auxiliary nurse, head for the bedside of an elderly patient, her tired pale blue eyes gazing vacantly ahead.

"Your friend has just rang to say she's coming to see you tomorrow."

"No, I don't want a bedpan thank you."

Slightly louder, the nurse repeated the sentence. "No, I said, your friend's coming to see you tomorrow. She's just rang."

"No I'm very comfortable thank you," said the patient.

The nurse bent over and adjusted Mrs Hudson's hearing aid and still talking quite loudly asked. "Can you hear me better now?"

"Stop shouting at me. You make my hearing aid vibrate."

The nurse gently said, "Your friends coming tomorrow."

"Pardon me, you'll have to speak up, I can't hear you."

Saturdays are devoid of all the hustle and bustle of week-days. Only the odd consultant checking on a patient or two. No cleaners, ladies after your blood or physio's after your body But this Saturday was different. We heard voices and laughter outside, suddenly a happy throng of wedding guests cascaded through the swing doors. The bride passed me in a summer cloud of tulle, followed by an effusion of pageboys and bridesmaids all heading for Violet. Customs and convention were ignored as the tiny bridesmaids excitedly spilled around the ward in a blur of pink. The joyous moments evaporated all too soon, as the visitors disappeared in a tumble of laughter, leaving the bouquet of peach and white roses for the proud Grandma.

The ward was awash with appreciative patients, even the ones in discomfort had been captivated and it had undoubtedly boosted everyone's morale. Well nearly everyone. Edna, a patient not renowned for her patience and understanding was not contributing to the excitement.

A nurse went over to her and asked. "Don't you think they all looked beautiful?"

There was a long pause, then with a long sigh and a shrug of resignation she muttered. " I suppose it was quite nice."

High praise indeed.

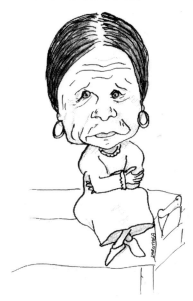

A nurse recalled the time they had two elderly patients who were in adjacent beds.

"They hated each other," said Vicky, "and the staff spent a great deal of time keeping them from doing each other a mischief. One had a gastric problem and needed specially prepared meals, such as steamed fish. When she saw her neighbour tucking into such things as fried fish and chips, she would become very aggressive and picking up her stick, would try and knock the other patients plate onto the floor. We tried to reason with her, but all she would say was, `don't blame me, its not my fault, its yours for giving me muck to eat.` I couldn't really argue with her," said Vicky.

Angela said she'd told a patient he had to have complete bedrest and could only use a commode by his bed if he wanted the loo. "He asked me for a commode and I duly wheeled it in place and drew the curtains leaving him to it. I was walking nearby when I noticed his head above the curtain rail. I rushed in to see what was happening. He was only standing on his bed and trying to pee into the commode from a great height. 'What are you doing?' I asked him. He looked at me in amazement. 'You told me I had to stay in bed,' he said. Well it was logical wasn't it?

The House Doctor was questioning a pale, wrinkly faced old lady. You know the sort, they look as if they've been left in the water too long.
"How far could you walk when you were well?" he asked.
"I could go to the shops."
"How far are the shops?"
"Just past the post box."
I heard a discernible sigh, but he persevered.
"How many yards do you think it is from your front door to the shops?"
There was a short silence, then I heard a small frail voice say.
"Oh, doctor, it must have been quite a way."
End of questioning.

"The only time I cried in twenty five years," said a staff nurse at Castle Hill, "was when a 76 year old Quaker had been diagnosed as having cancer. I already knew that in the last year alone she had lost an eight year old grandson, her mother, two

54

sisters, and a close friend, all with the disease. She said to me, `Don't worry, its all right. Its God's way.` She had an implicit faith which you could almost reach out and touch."

One of the ever lasting memories will be the sight of a fourteen stone, 69 year old, parading through the ward, her scarlet lip-stick escaping in small rivulets into the white floury face powder, shifting the course of her real mouth. She was dressed in a short see-through nightie, her sagging boobs flapped happily against the protruding tum, which was encased in long white knickers, doing nothing to disguise the fact that underneath she was wearing large blue incontinence pads.

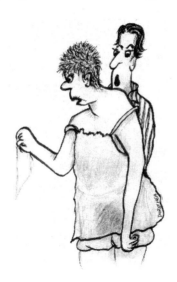

At the end of the ward were two toilets, for patients' use only and we had two older ladies who liked to commandeer them for long periods of time. The nurses would wheel them down in wheelchaisr and they were instructed to pull the red cord when they'd finished. Half-an-hour later a nurse would go to investigate. "No, we're all right." they insisted. An hour later there were at least three desperate patients seeking relief in the lavatory. Dorothy came reasonably quietly but Bella was not so forthcoming. They had to physically pull her off the seat and return her to bed.

Six am and the ward was coming to after a rather stressful night. An elderly lady in a flowered dressing gown suddenly appeared at the side of my bed. She had a strange shadow all around her hair-line, caused, I guessed, by the dye from black hair colorant.

"Hello," she said.

"Hello," I replied.

"Do you know where I'm going?" she asked.

"Where do you want to go?"

"Well I'd like to go to bed."

"Well just go through that door and you'll see lady in a striped dress. She'll tell you where to go."

She smiled, patted my hand and toddled off.

I looked towards a sprightly seventy year old who had been admitted the previous day wearing a dark brown wig, perched perilously on her head with tendrils of white peeping out, framing her chubby, weather beaten face. She had not removed the wig to go to sleep and during the night it had slid beautifully over her left ear. I promise you it was a sight to behold.

Further down the ward I saw a patient suddenly climb out of bed. He stood to attention and started to slap himself very hard - all over - he missed nothing out! "To get the circulation going." he declared. "After this I'm ready for the world and those bloody nurses."

In the bed next to me lay Daisy, an elderly, doughty Yorkshire woman She also had been watching our five foot six Rambo. "Silly bugger." she said dismissively

Daisy commented on everything. When her tea was a little short on milk, she would call out, "What's up lass, has coo run dry?"

If she dropped something on the floor, it invariably was followed by, "Damn, I've dropped my, biscuit/glasses/ etc. on the dog shelf."

She told me one day, "My elder sister's coming to see me today."

"Elder sister? But you're 94."

"Yes, that's right. Our Mildred, she's 96, but our Herbert's 98. Mildred's the one living."

I'd worked that out for myself unless she had a direct phone-line to you-know-who!

I heard all about her daughter and the problems she'd had in pregnancy.

"Oohh, you'll nivver believe it," she said, "but our Josephine had a stone born baby you know."

I looked suitably aghast.

When you're bedbound, talkative patients can be a real pain - if you'll excuse the pun - Charlie was one such body. He would target his prey and head off, his zimmer frame klonking along at a rate of knots. I saw him talking to a patient who didn't want to talk to him. Charlie had somehow got his zimmer stuck in the bedside table. He pulled and yanked and all he managed to do was tip the water jug over the protesting patient. Two nurses came to lead him back to his bed. There was a nurse on either side to assist, but this 79 year old did not want to return to bed. He pushed and shoved with such insistence, in the direction he wanted to go, that everyone ended up in the day room. So they let him stay.

Talking about zimmer frames reminds me of a guy on the ward who'd had a hip replacement. The day before he was due to be released a nurse saw him strolling down the ward with a zimmer frame over his shoulder.

"Why are you carrying the frame on your shoulder?" asked Gloria.

"The physio said I had to."

"Had to what?"

"Said I shouldn't go anywhere without it."

It was three am and Annie felt the need to visit the loo. She returned to find Maude in her bed. I called the nurse who came and led Maude back to her bed. The following night I was sound asleep when I was aware of being pushed. Maude had returned, but this time she was trying to tip me out so she could climb in. I'm pleased to say they put up the side guards on her bed after that."

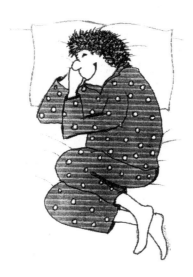

Maud wasn't the only one to go walkabout. A couple of nights later I heard Violet asking if anyone had seen her glasses.

"Where did you leave them?" asked the nurse.

"On my bedside cabinet."

They searched all around but no glasses were found.

"What did they look like?

"No frames, just a gold nose bridge and side ear pieces. But the top half of the lenses were coloured."

The nurse frowned, but said nothing. Ten minutes later she returned holding out a pair of spectacles. "Are these yours?"

"Yes," said a delighted Violet. "Where did you find them?"

"Sorry, but it was Marjorie. During the night she went to the loo and on the way took a fancy to your specs. She was sat up in bed wearing them. Couldn't see a thing mind you."

I guessed we were in for one of those days. I saw an auxiliary heading for Staff Nurse Sally. "Ward eighteen have lost some teeth, they wondered if we had any extras."

"Can't say I've noticed a spare set hanging around." she replied.

"Well a patient said the woman who was brought to you from ward eighteen, took his teeth."

They went over to the new arrival. "Gwen have you got an extra set of teeth?"

Gwen looked suitably surprised, then took out her dentures, solemnly surveyed them, popped them back and told them, "No, these are definitely mine." Sally was just turning away, when Gwen continued: "My husband keeps his in a drawer at home. He won't wear them, so if that man wants he can borrow George's."

An elderly lady had been admitted to the ward and I heard the nurse ask her to undress, telling her she would return in a few minutes.

From behind the curtains I heard a strangulated "Nurse," so pressed my emergency button. Cynthia came immediately. I pointed to the next bed and told her it was the new patient. The nurse was with her for nearly twenty minutes, while the most horrific sounds came from behind the curtain.

Evidently she was wearing a roll-on, one of those elasticised contraptions that were supposed to flatten your tum, but this time it had shot up like a demented roller blind and nestled around her waist in a vice-like grip.

"She looked as if she was being strangled." said the nurse.

"The wretched thing seemed to be getting tighter. She couldn't have been in more trouble if she'd been engulfed by a giant boa-constrictor. Eventually I decided the only thing I could do was cut her free. I cut through the elastic very carefully as I was convinced the thing would react violently if it came undone too quickly. I could see the headlines: "Patient wins fight for life with a girdle"'

Now that would be original.

I was telling Nurse Hughes the story and it reminded her of another scissors story. She told me: "An elderly patient was being discharged and he'd had a catheter inserted." said Kath. "As he was getting ready to leave I noticed him fiddling around his waist band, so went to ask what he was doing, then realised he had a pair of scissors in his hand. He'd only cut through the tube and was putting the bag of urine in his shopping carrier. 'It's easier like this' he told me."

Like Kath said. "There's nowt so queer as folk."


I was feeling a bit sorry for myself when I heard the following conversation between the indomitable Staff Nurse Cathy and a patient at Castle Hill Hospital.

Patient: I've got cystitis, what can you give me?

Nurse: We don't give medication, but Lemon Barley does the trick.

Patient: I haven't got any.

Nurse: Don't worry, I'll go and pinch some from one of the other patients.

Patient: You can't do that.

Nurse: Course I can. Especially for someone who brags like you.

Patient: Me, bragging?

Nurse: Well you know it's the honeymooner's disease, don't you?

Patient: Honeymooner's disease? You've got to be joking. I'm 69.

Nurse: Now you know what I mean about the bragging!

Off she went, returning a few minutes later with a bottle of Lemon Barley.

Margaret popped into see an auntie of hers who had just been discharged from hospital after being diagnosed as diabetic.

She was still having a few problems, mainly with headaches and nausea. The hospital had given her a weeks supply of pills which had to be taken twice a day.

Margaret noticed a pill bottle in the kitchen and it appeared full.

"Are these your new pills?" she asked.

"No, they're the ones the doctor gave me last week."

That's what I meant. But the bottle is still full, aren't you taking them?"

"Oh, yes," replied Auntie Kath. "They're marvellous, so I'm keeping a few back in case they won't give me any more."

# THE WORLD
## ACCORDING TO LOUISA

As you can see, during my numerous visits to hospital I have met many wonderful characters. Many of the oldies were enchanting, none more that 82 year old Louisa. She was an absolute joy. Five foot one of pure femininity. She had lived life to the full and still retained an indomitable spirit which was palpable. She had, as Terry Wogan would say, 'some senior moments,' but these made her even more endearing. I made notes constantly and have devoted a whole chapter to that very special lady.

I hope you find her as entertaining as I did.

She used to pad around the ward in a china blue dressing gown, perfectly matching her twinkling blue eyes. She had delicate, doll like features, framed by silver curly hair. She'd already had both knees replaced, a hip and a shoulder. "The muscles have gone in the other shoulder," she told me "and I'm told I really need instant surgery, but the doctor told me he hadn't got any money for shoulders, but then said he loved operating on shoulders, they were his very, very favourites, so he was sure he would be able to get some cash from somewhere."

"When did he tell you that?"

"Oh, that was two years ago. But you have to keep cheerful don't you?"

Every day Louisa would wash out a pair of knickers - pink,

edged with a wisp of frivolous white lace- hanging them out to dry in the most bizarre places.

TUESDAY

She had spied a redundant zimmer frame and hung her daily wash over the top. Diane the physio came striding over: "Whose are these?" she asked. Louisa confessed. Diane returned them to her. Undeterred, Louisa draped them across an empty flower vase.

Tea-time and a nurse saw Louisa polishing her cutlery.

"What are you doing Louisa?"

"Cleaning my knives and forks."

"But we clean them really thoroughly here."

"Not clean enough for me. So I'm cleaning them again."

"What are you cleaning them with?"

"My knickers."

WEDNESDAY

Louisa applied make-up every morning. Today she came trotting from the bathroom, newly washed knickers draped over her arm, when a nurse made a comment on her underwear.

"Why is it you noticed my knickers, but never said a word about my new lipstick? I bet you'd never say anything to my friend Doris either. She always looks after herself and never goes out without her going out teeth in."

As Amanda said, "There's not a lot you can say to that."

The day had dawned bright and sunny so the knickers were taken outside and draped over a green plastic chair, but there was quite a strong wind and they were soon whisked onto the ground. Smiling sweetly, she approached an elderly male visitor: "Could you please pick up my laundry, it seems to have fallen off the chair?" The man obliged, bent to pick them up and only then realised he was holding knickers. They were dropped swiftly onto the bed and he made a hasty retreat. I heard Louisa mutter: "Oh heck, I'll now have ants in me pants."

I had no visitors that afternoon so Louisa came padding over and sat on my bed. We were discussing life in general when she leant over conspiratorially and whispered: "Have you seen that woman over there in the yellow nightie?"

I peeped over in her direction and nodded.

"Have you seen the amount of chocolates she puts away?"

I had to admit I hadn't noticed anything untoward.

"Well, It's a wonder she isn't the size of a barrage balloon. If she sat next to a fire she'd melt." and with that padded away.

## THURSDAY

Several of the patients were discussing smoking and Louisa gave us her words of wisdom:

"Why stop smoking, it takes ten to fifteen years to clear your lungs and you'll probably be dead by then anyway."

Later that morning a Red Cross volunteer came to change the flowers, she headed for Louisa's bed. "These could do with throwing away," she told her. "Is that all right, or shall I leave then a bit longer?"

"Oh throw them away. Anyway it's germs in the water that kills cut flowers?"

"Oh, I don't know about that. I mean some have been here for two weeks."

"There you are then. They've died because of the germs."

The Red Cross lady didn't argue and asked her if she knew when she might be going home.

"Oh, soon," said Louisa. "And when I get out of here I think I'll treat myself to a music stand to put all my things on."

"That's a good idea."

"Mmmm, I've been thinking. I'm going to get one of those telescopic ones that zoom up and down."

I had wonderful visions of the stand, whooshing up and down and being completely out of control in the delicate hands of this fragrant lady.

Later in the afternoon we were discussing ages and how

difficult it was in these modern times to tell a person's age.

Louisa told us. "My niece is 32, she only looks 30, it's in the genes you know She's a funny girl, her mind jumps from one thing to another as if she's nothing else to do. She works in a charity shop you know. Mind you their Billy is another funny one. He always brings his dog when he visits. He lets it outside and it does it's," she shuddered, and paused for a moment. "Well you know, shit!" I never thought the word would pass her lips, but she carried on "I swear the silly animal holds it all in 'till he gets to my house. No wonder he's got a fat stomach. If I see him coming I rush to put the clocks on an hour. He's never noticed yet."

I think she was talking about Billy not the dog!

*FRIDAY*
The doctor was on his rounds and stopped by Louisa's bed. He was checking her files, then asked about her knee.

"Are you going to protestigate?"

"Sorry." said the doctor, "What do you mean?"

"Are you going to have a look round?"

"Ahh!" a smile crossed his face. "No, I don't think we'll need to investigate your knee again Louisa."

After lunch, she was holding forth on gardens and was telling the staff nurse that she had planted some, "really pretty flowers before I came in here."

"Did you?" asked Cathy, "How unusual, I only put ugly ones in mine."

"Now you're being silly," she told her.

Visitors were strewn around the ward and a very pretty three year old girl, her blonde hair tied in bunches framing a chubby, smiling face, was sat on the floor near her Grandma's bed. Louisa called out to her. "Do you know, you look just like a little frog."

The mother and proud grandmother looked suitably aghast at this remark. Louisa was quite unaware of their dismay and went on to explain: "It's her big eyes and the way she's sitting on the floor. They do that you know. Always with their head held high."

It's a good job Grandma was discharged the next day as she was not best pleased with our Louisa.

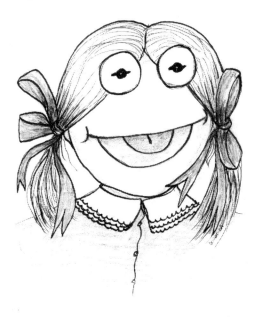

SATURDAY

"Have I told you about my neighbour?"

"Don't think so." I said.

"She eats like nobody I've ever seen. Ooohh, I wish I could eat like her. Do you know she can eat a duck. She's 89 and eats mountains and usually at eight o'clock at night and the milkman wont deliver her milk she's so horrid. I tell you if she gets to heaven there's hope for me yet." She turned and busied herself tidying up her cupboard. She suddenly looked up and saw Barbara walking past her bed pushing her drip in front of her. Louisa called out. "Lovely day for a wander and it's nice to see you're taking your dog for a walk again."

A visitor came into the ward in a motorised wheelchair and Louisa went over for a chat and inspection of the vehicle. She told the lady:

"When I get out I'm going to get one of those three wheeler cars."

"Do you mean a Robin Reliant?"

"No, no, no. These are much smaller wheels, except my shed door isn't big enough. If somebody would knock it down I could get one in."

"But if you knock it down you wont have a shed," said a bemused lady.

"No, no, no, I mean knock down the doors. I've also got a coal bunker, but that's full of baskets. I can drive you know and a scooter would be very nice indeed." And with that wandered back to her bed.

## SUNDAY

"Did you know my binman has got two degrees?" she said to no-one in particular. "That's it you see, they come out with an armful of rolled up degrees and silly hats and think they know it all."

"I thought you said he was a binman."

"He is. That's it you see. He's totally happy. He could have saved all that silly learning and done it from the beginning. That's real happiness you know. I dont think the silly hats help, do you?"

The paperman scurried in on his daily round and Louisa bought one of every magazine he had.

"You must like reading." he said.

"Oh, they're not for me," said Louisa. "I'll take them home and give them to old people."

At 82, she obviously considered herself only middle-aged.

## MONDAY

A porter came into the ward with a wheelchair to take a patient to x-ray but she was receiving treatment behind the curtains, so while waiting, he made himself comfortable in the chair.

Louisa looked up from her bed and called out. "What are you doing in the girls dormitory?"

He smiled mischievously and beckoning to her said: "I'm a doctor, trust me and come and sit on my knee."

"I will do nothing of the kind." said a shocked Louisa. "I'm not frightened of people like you any more. I was ten years in the airforce and they taught me everything. Oh yes, I could tell you a thing or two and I'd take you on anytime."

"I take it you're not going to sit on my knee then."

Before she had time to answer the curtains opened and Mrs Chadwick appeared ready to be taken for her x-ray.

When they'd gone, Louisa proceeded to tell us about her friends.

"We always meet, once a week, all eight of us, six ladies and two men. We've all been in the forces, so we have a real good laugh and we talk a lot, that's really just to stop Clarice going on because all her family are brain surgeons, rocket scientists or nuclear physic. thingys."

"And as for Edwin, he knows everything, but if truth be told you could write in capital letters all he knows on the belly-button of a flea. We also go quite a lot to the theatre. I love the ballet, we've paid as much as £37. That was for the Russians. But oh, dear what a disappointment. They were all dressed in black and all we saw was silly gymnastics. Now the Scottish Opera are always worth seeing. We pay £33 for them. Mind you the last time they came the tickets were £35 and they were only doing Carmen. Now if it had been a famous opera, but who wants to pay good money to watch a silly woman in a red dress prancing about."

I swear she told this story without taking breath.

*TUESDAY*

A German doctor came to check on Louisa.

"I see you're up and walking." he said.

"Yes that's right. I do what I can."

"Yes. That is good. You are one of the better well people."

"Better well! Better well! How can I be better well if I'm still in here?" fumed Louisa.

A local photographer had requested an old person to photograph for a selection of pictures he was planning showing the ageing process. The hospital selected Louisa. Several patients were waiting in the day room when in strode the photographer, a young boy trailing behind carrying all the equipment. Louisa was resplendent in a smart silk blouse, eye-shadow and lipstick, all ready for her big moment, but the photographer walked straight past her. He asked sister where was the old lady they had come to photograph. She pointed to Louisa. The photographer gasped. "Good God, that's not what we want at all. We want an old woman."

"But she is 82," said sister.

"She might be 82, but who expects women of that age to wear make-up? Haven't you got anyone else?"

"Only ones who are too poorly to get out of bed."

"Oh scrub it then. I'll try somewhere else."

With that he turned on his heel and walked out.

Excitement over, most of the patients shuffled back to their beds, headed by a disgruntled Louisa. She first sat in her chair then called out. "I'm going to have a lie-down." She had only been settled for a few minutes when she suddenly sat bolt upright and announced that she'd like her bedside light on.

"Don't call a nurse," said Maria, "I'll do it for you.".

"Oh thank you. You'll find two switches behind my bed, well, just press one down."

"Which one do I press?" asked Maria.

"The other one." informed Louisa.

"Which other one?"

Louisa tutted rather loudly and with a great sigh told her: "Not the one you shouldn't."

WEDNESDAY
"Have you wet the bed?" asked Staff nurse Cathy.

"Certainly not." said a very indignant Louisa.

"I bet you have."

"When I do that I know I'll have reached old age."

"Go on," said Cathy, "I do it. It keeps you warm in winter."

Later in the morning, Cathy came round with the drug trolley. Louisa looked suspiciously into the receptacle she'd just been given.

"How many have I got?"

"Three."

"What are they?" persisted Louisa.

"Arsenic, Bromide and Viagra." said Cathy.

"Did you know you can't buy arsenic any more?"

"Can't you?" asked Cathy.

"No, I tried several places, but they wouldn't let me have any."

"They're saving it all for me." replied Cathy

Louisa giggled and took the pills, then laid back, closed her eyes and went soundly to sleep.

In the afternoon it was Staff Nurse Amanda who was doling out the medication.

"Do you know what Cathy told me these pills were?" she asked.

"No, surprise me."

Louisa thought for a moment then triumphantly announced, "Arsenic, Bromide and Velcro."

"Wow," exclaimed Amanda. "Did they do you any good?"

"Not really, I wish she hadn't given me them."

"Why's that then?"

"Because they seem to make my whistling worse."

Amanda didn't question this remark but I was dying to know more.

The nurses came round the ward selling tombola tickets while I was away having an X-ray. When I returned, Louisa told me: "I hope you don't mind, but I got you a trombola ticket."

Wonder if it was a musical charity?

*THURSDAY*

Louisa had a bed next to the wide windows, which overlooked a large grassed area. "Have you seen the blackbirds trying to pull out the worms?" she asked me.

I admitted I had.

"The little worms don't stand a chance do they?".

"Oh I don't know," I said, "they can wriggle pretty quick."

"But have you seen the size of those birds? They'd make a lovely dinner for four. I think I'll try and nab one before I go and stick it in my freezer for Christmas. If a King can bake them in a pie, I'm sure they'll be lovely roasted. Wonder if I should have mint, apple or cranberry sauce with them?"

"Can't help you with that one Louisa, sorry."

With a twinkle she said, "I wonder what worm sauce tastes like?"

A student nurse was asking Louisa about her family and she told her, her daughter was a 'high flyer' in the city. "If you want to ring her up just say and I can bring the phone to your bedside." said the student.

"Oh, no thank you," said Louisa, "I'm not sure where she'll be and you wont catch me leaving messages with a tin man."

She went on to tell us that when her daughter got married, she couldn't find a pair of shoes that were the right colour.

"I soon sorted it though. I scrubbed an old pair with washing up liquid, then I emulsioned them with the prettiest shade of pink you ever saw. Nobody noticed a thing. Mind you I always ask a cobbler to put a thing on my heel. That stops me going backwards."

*FRIDAY*

The night had been particularly noisy and when the nurses came round with breakfast they first asked if everyone had slept well. Louisa called out. "No I didn't. But then I never do. Once when I came into hospital, I didn't sleep a wink for five days, so when

I got home I slept the sleep of the dead. But my husband was so concerned he kept waking me up to see if I was all right."

"Sounds like my husband, but he's only after sex," muttered a nurse.

Louisa's eyes opened and she exclaimed: "Ooh, that's naughty."

"Never mind about my love life, or lack of it, what do you want for breakfast?"

"A Weetabix please."

"Just one?"

"Oh yes, I think so." replied Louisa. "I used to eat four, but that was in the days I played football for England."

Who says when you're a wrinklie you lose your sense of humour.

We'd all finished our breakfast and were waiting for a cup of tea. Suddenly out of the blue Louisa started chattering.

"I used to go to art class," she told no-one in particular. "but I'm afraid they kicked me out, mainly for giggling and not taking it seriously. It came to a head when we were asked to draw a tree. I didn't fancy that so I drew a bird, but my bird was hanging upside down from a telegraph pole. That was a tree wasn't it? My bird had two beaks and three legs. 'You have something,' the tutor told me, but he didn't know what. Actually I agreed and went home to rummage."

I think she meant ruminate.

By ten o'clock the ward was a hive industry with nurses, doctors, cleaners and the ubiquitous phlebotomists. Louisa as usual started chatting and told Sue: "I think my friend Annie's coming to see me today."

"That's nice. Where's she coming from?"

"From where she lives." replied Louisa.

"Where's that?"

"Where her house is of course. She's a very nice lady but sometimes she gets so excited her petticoats start trembling."

Now that's what I call excitement!

72

The rest of the day passed reasonably quietly until the evening drugs round and the nurse asked Louisa what she'd had for tea.

"Mushrooms and custard."

"Mushrooms and custard?"

"Oh yes, didn't you see it. I saved mine to show my friend." She leant over and opened her bedside cabinet bringing out a small white plastic container. Inside were the remnants of her tea. It was bananas and custard but the fruit had gone decidedly black and the nurse admitted it looked exactly like mushrooms and custard.

"I've just thought," said Louisa, "I wonder if they have a scientifical laboratory here, they'd probably be very interested."

After the drug round Louisa would carry out her daily ritual. Sitting on the edge of her bed, she would solemnly dunk a curler into her water jug and proceed to roll up her hair. Curlers were placed neatly in a row around her face. The back was never touched. Each morning it was all carefully combed out, with the back remaining a tangled riot of silver. "You have to look after yourself," she told us, "You never know who you might meet."

SATURDAY
"Did you have a good nights sleep Louisa?"

"I did not. It was like sleeping in the middle of a factory with all those buzzers going off." She then toddled off to the bathroom, giving me a wave on the way. When she returned, damp knickers dangling over her left arm, she stopped by my bed and out of the blue asked if I could drive. I nodded.

"I can drive you know."

"Can you?"

"Mmmm. Ooh, it was years ago that I learnt to drive." she sighed deeply. "But they never gave me a licence you know."

"Why's that Louisa?"

"Because I could never remember which pedal I should put my feet on." and without drawing breath continued, "and a friend of mine refuses to get in a car with her daughter."

73

"Why not?"

"She just wont. She gets really distraughted at her driving."

She then carefully re-arranged her knickers over her arm - I did think for a minute she was going to leave them with me - but she turned and returned to her bed.

In the afternoon two ladies came to visit Louisa and stayed for some time chatting away. When they'd gone I remarked "You looked like you were having a good old chin-wag."

"Oh yes, we did, but do you know what they told me?" She was shaking her head sadly. "I have a mobile hairdresser who comes to see me when I'm at home and they only told me David was in hospital. I told them, I hope he doesn't die yet, who will do my hair when I get out?"

Louisa was a font of knowledge on old superstitions but seemed to find the most in-opportune moments to impart her nuggets of wisdom.

I had been admitted with a pulmonary embolism and was finding even shallow breathing exceedingly painful, so could not hold long conversations. I had told friends and relatives not to visit, just send a funny card telling me all the latest gossip, but I wasn't too worried when I saw Louisa toddling my way, although she could chat for England she hardly ever expected, or waited for a reply.

She patted my hand. "Don't worry if you can't afford a hot-water bottle," she told me, "Just take some pages of newspaper or magazines and put them in the oven for a while. Make sure you lift up some of the pages so the hot air can circulate. Then put them in an old nightie and they'll keep you warm for hours."

"Ooh!" she exclaimed and pointed to my hands. "You have rheumatism don't you? Well I know a wonderful cure." She was now in full flow: "Mix some camphor and mentholated spirits and put it on the affected part. My friend Millie said she used it regularly and it cured her mother."

I knew I could rely on Louisa to perk me up. She paused only for a moment then asked: "Did you know you should never dig up a parsley root and give it to a friend? I shook my head. "Oh yes, " she said. "If she wants it she has to dig it up herself. My mother told me a friend of hers did and she fell down dead the next day and the other fell and broke her glasses."

I looked suitably concerned then she suddenly asked if I had a garden. "Mmm." I muttered, wondering what was coming next. "And you're married aren't you?"

"Mmm." Now it was getting interesting.

"Well if you boil some ivy leaves in a pan, you can use the liquid to take all those shiny bits off your husband's suits."

I thought I'd show willing and asked if I should just dab it or soak the whole area.

"Oh, as you please. Are you going to try it then?"

"Well, you never know, I might."

She patted my hand and smiling brightly completely changed the subject by asking "Have you ever owned a business?" I nodded. "Well let me tell you something," she said. "If the first person in your shop comes in without buying anything, you'll have a really bad week, so the best thing is, go outside and come back in pretending to be a customer and purchase something, even if it's only a beetroot."

I had a slight problem. I owned a travel shop!

# FOOD

In the time of mixed wards I was put in bed next to Ernie, who loved anything that could be stuffed into his mouth. He was continually belching. He would pat his over-sized stomach and inform everybody. "Perfect. Sign of a bloody good meal that."

In ward nine, ladies who were not bedbound were asked to be seated in the centre of the ward for meals.

Every mealtime Doris would ceremoniously, liberally douse her wrists before she joined the other patients.

One day a frail seventy-seven year old piped up. "I wish you wouldn't come to the table with that Estee Lauder."

"What are you talking about," asked Doris, " I don't know any Estee Lauder, who's Estee lauder?"

I nearly choked on my boiled cabbage. She wasn't joking.

As the nurses busied themselves serving lunch to the patients, I heard Maureen ask: "Are you ready for your rice pudding yet Kathleen?"

"No, not yet, another couple of minutes. I like it hot." replied Kathleen.

When they brought it a few minutes later, the nurse cleared her tray and planting the dish of rice pudding firmly in the middle said," There you are. Sorry it's not hot, just a bit warm around the edges."

"But I told you I like it hot."

"I know but we had extra ice-cream so thought we'd treat

you and plonk some on top."

It didn't improve by tea-time, when the nurse opened the doors to start dishing out the meals, she found they'd put the jellies in the oven, but they battled on checking lists and taking the relevant meal to the patients..

"There's your tea Muriel."

"What is it?"

"Cottage pie."

"Cottage pie. What's that?"

"Mince and mash with baked beans."

"I don't want that. I only have sausages with baked beans."

"Well you ordered it."

"Well you can un-order it. Unless I can have sausages.."

"They only come with liver."

"I want them with baked beans."

"Well you can't."

"All right. What's for pudding?"

"Cheese custard or fruit yoghurt."

"Uuugghh! Cheese and custard."

"No Muriel, not cheese and custard. Cheese custard."

"It sounds stupid to me, so does that other thing you said. I'm not chancing it. I'll only have pudding."

She left Muriel and went to try and persuade an elderly patient to eat her dinner.

"Come on Minnie, you can eat more than that."

"Why have you changed my name? I'm Ada."

"You mean you don't know?"

"No."

"`cos you're a moaning Minnie, that's why."

Which reminds me of the previous day when two ladies who were squaring up to each other.

"I 'ate 'aving lettuce." said Maude.

"Do you mean let us alone?" queried Sally.

"No, you silly sod, with something."

"Well why don't you say lettiss, instead of let-us, then?"

"I can say what I bloody well like, so just let us alone."

The perfect repartee and they didn't have a clue how comic it had been.

The following day we were waiting eagerly for our lunch, well as eagerly as you can for hospital food, but I'd ordered shepherd's pie and apple crumble, two of my favourites.

The trolley's were wheeled ceremoniously into the ward, the plates taken out and all the nurses were stood expectantly by. With a flourish sister opened the doors. Every shelf was empty. They'd forgotten to put in any food. When they eventually returned the only thing the kitchen had left was left was fish and chips. Have you ever tried slightly warm fish and chips? Suddenly that cheese sandwich my son had left the night before became irresistible. Even with the curled corners!

After lunch a patient called out: "Nurse I've finished. Bring my dessert now."

"You're not at the Ritz now you know" called the nurse.

"No," said the patient, "But I've finished, so I'd like my dessert."

The nurse went over to her, curtsied right down to the ground and said, "Your Majesty. I do apologise. But you'll bloody wait like everyone else."

Gladys Whitaker was a patient in the hospital and watched as a family of seven would come to visit Big Doris every night, laden with Chinese take-aways.

"Big Doris?!"

"Yes, that's right. They would draw the curtains round the bed and tuck in. The smell stayed for hours. Oh and then there was Peggy. She was a large pale faced woman who wore quite the scruffiest nightie you've ever seen. After her family had gone she would sit and eat the delicacies they'd brought her. Winkles."

"Winkles?"

"Yes, winkles. She would pull the eye off and throw it on the floor. She would devour the little worm thing and the shell would be tossed under her bed. Except it was a polished floor and winkle shells were skidding everywhere. She was told to stop it, but she took not a blind bit of notice."

This reminded me of Albert who loved peanuts. His family brought him bags full, all with their shells on. He would crack them open and casually toss the shells on the floor. "I don't know how he sleeps," said a nurse, "because every time we make his bed, it's littered with discarded husks."

But even I had to admit neither of these were a patch on Big Doris.

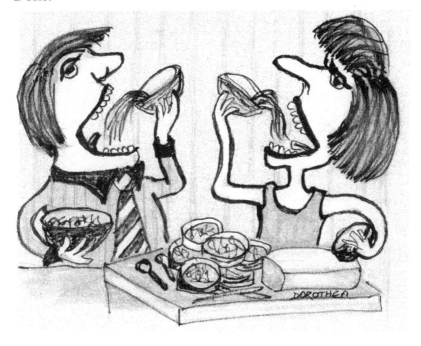

# FUNEREAL

I remember being intrigued by a headline which asked: "How do you live to be a hundred?"

The answer? "Stay away from funerals - especially your own."

They also say that the only two things you can't escape in life is income tax and your own funeral.

Which I suppose is pretty accurate and I know someone who would have probably agreed with those comments.

I was holidaying near Granada in Spain and was rather taken aback by a story in a newspaper. Evidently the local mayor of Lanjarun, had banned any of the residents from dropping dead because the towns one graveyard had space for only six more people.

Mr Gonzalez urged residents "Go to the doctor's if you feel ill and eat the right food. If you die from now ( 1st Oct. 1999 ) you'll be breaking the law and your family will have to pay a fine."

If you think that's bizarre, a landlord in Saddleworth, near Oldham in Lancashire, decided to open a graveyard in the back garden of his boozer.

Enterprising Julian Taylor realised that all the graveyards nearby were full and the field behind his pub had room for at least 2,500 graves - and it could end up making more money than selling beer.

Each plot has room for a family of four and the going rate at the moment is £1000. He advertised: "His and hearse graves." Obviously a man with a sense of humour. He managed to get planning permission after asking his local vicar to bless the site.

The landlord admitted he hoped the graveyard would bring in more business. "Relatives who bury their loved ones in the garden can retire to my pub for the wake."

He offered cut price rates for the first few weeks and the first to stump up was pub regular Trevor Booth.

The 57 year old stone-wall repairer has a stake marked No 1 into his cut price plot. "It's the grave nearest the pub," said Trevor, "It'll be nice to lie out the back with the smell of booze wafting over you."

His drinking companion joined in: "I like the idea of drinking a pint in my favourite pub and looking at where I'll be at the end of my days."

There was not a dissenting voice. Even the undertaker thought it was, "A brilliant idea. The location is ideal. Some mourners don't fancy a long drive to the bar after they've buried a relative."

I've just thought, I bet some relatives will be there to offer an ale and farewell to friends and relatives or maybe they'll only be there for the bier - sorry about that - but either way, it'll probably make more money than selling bottles of Boddingtons!

In the 1800's there was a man called Cyfartha who owned a large iron works in Wales, he programmed his funeral down to the last detail. He even chose and supervised the cutting of the wood for his coffin.

He had three requests. One, that only one person should be in the cortege car, and that should be the conductor of his renowned, works brass band. His coffin should be in a grave exactly fourteen feet deep and it was to be covered by a stone no less that five tons in weight.

I was on a long week-end in the beautiful city of Dublin and was rather intrigued at a notice in a funeral parlour's window. "Funerals arranged. Self-drive available."

While in Poland a cortege was clustered around a grave, saying their farewells to a loved one, when they heard the muffled, but distinctive sound of a mobile phone, coming from the next grave in which a man had only been interred the previous day. Two ladies fainted and three mourners ran away screaming.

A friend of mine spent his life driving fast cars. He particularly enjoyed rally driving. When he passed away he left a memo for his wife. It read: "Under no circumstances do I want the hearse to go at the accepted pace, tell them to go as fast as the speed limit allows."
The problem was, no-one-one had told the mourners and they couldn't understand why they were all going like a bat out of hell along Hessle Road.

Tony Richards was an ambulance driver and his regular colleague was off sick, so he had another ambulanceman to share the duties for one day only. Tony was renowned for odd things happening to him while on duty. "You name it, I've experienced it," he said. "I think the only thing I never did was deliver twins at the top of a flagpole but I've been near a couple of times." He laughed. "I remember one particular day when we were called to an area off Holderness Road. As we turned into the street I noticed banners and balloons strung across the road and a lot of happy people. A street party was in full swing and the ambulance was led through the revellers to a house at the end of the street. We were ushered up the stairs of a small terrace house and into the front bedroom. As soon as we checked we knew the gentleman had died. I decided to go back to the ambulance and call the station. I asked if they could get a doctor to come out and certify the patient dead at the scene. Half-an-hour went by and they said a doctor couldn't be found so we were instructed to take him straight to the mortuary. We didn't want to spoil the party outside so we put his teeth back in, popped his glasses on, then lifted him into a chair. Wrapping him up securely in a blanket, making sure it covered his head, looking like a comatose Father Christmas, we carried him down into the street. He was put in the ambulance with cries of, 'Chin up,' 'We'll bring you some grapes' and, 'don't worry Ted we'll look after the missus' ringing in our ears we drove away."

"It could only have happened to me." said Tony..

He also recalled the time an elderly lady had gassed herself. "When we arrived we noticed a note on the kitchen table. It said 'Please look after Joey the budgie. He's been my friend and would like him to go to a good home.' Problem was," said Mr Richards, "Poor old Joey was laid on the bottom of his cage, feet pointing stiffly heavenwards. He was in the same room as the gas oven so had expired quietly with his owner."

"Can't say the same for a gent. we went to pick up in a factory in Hull. It was about 9.00 pm and as we pulled up to the gates a distressed lady was stood in the middle of the road, she told us where we had to go but refused to come in with us. We made our way to the second floor, as directed, and entered a typical office with numerous desks and office equipment. We found a gentleman laid out on a blanket - dead. It was obvious what had been going on, so we put a blanket around the body and carried him on a stretcher to the ambulance. The lady was waiting and by now nearly hysterical. We told her 'don't worry, the gentleman will be fully dressed before we get him to hospital. None of his relatives will ever know, adding under my breath, ' that he died a happy man."

Which is not what I can say about a man who'd been cremated after he'd died. His widow couldn't decide what to do with the ashes. They were left for a while in the crematorium, then she eventually rang and asked for them to be released as 'she didn't want him left there with all those dead people.' She decided to put them under a rose tree, but the thing died. A very disgruntled lady told me I wouldn't mind but I had to dig him up again. I asked what she'd done with him. 'Oh, he's stuck in the pantry until I can afford another rose tree."

I am not normally a nervous individual, but I must admit I do feel pretty apprehensive when I'm in a small 'plane, while a storm is raging. I was on the runway in Barbados on a small 'Liat' flight to St. Lucia when suddenly the aircraft cut its engines and we were told to dis-embark. The engine was malfunctioning they said. We changed planes and as I nervously sat waiting for take-off clearance I recalled a pilot once telling me, that a good method to decrease stress and anxiety is to engage in conversation, so I turned to the man sitting alongside me. "Hello, I'm Dorothea. Are you as nervous as me?" The tall, gangly, stranger turned, smiled and held out a hand. "Hi, I'm Geoff. and no I'm not. Would you feel better if I hold your hand?" I nodded enthusiastically. "Are you here on holiday?" He shook his head. "What do you do for a living?" I asked. He turned and with a huge grin replied: "I'm an undertaker and you'll never guess what my surname is, Berriman!"

Funeral directors have to be a special sort of person. I remember one telling me that he never thought in a million years he'd be able to do a job like that. "But it's a funny old world," he told me. "after only three days, I thought it was easy. Except for the time I saw a man get run over by a train at Paragon Station. We had to sort him out. We were picking him up all over the place. `I've nivver seen owt like it in me life."

He saw me pull a face and said "It's not all doom and gloom you know, sometimes you can have a right laugh. I mean there was the time we were motoring sedately along to the crematorium, followed by the funeral party. We were just entering the gates on Chanterlands Avenue when the hearse started to slow down, then did a wonderful impression of a kangaroo. The rest of the cavalcade also slowed thinking we must be running out of petrol. Suddenly our driver realised he was on the wrong bloody tank so quickly switched over. We spluttered back to life and continued uneventfully up the driveway. The waiting congregation were more than a little surprised when all the funeral party climbed out of their car giggling uncontrollably.

"Whatever's happened?" asked a relative.

They explained about the wayward hearse and added: "Grandma always said she would only go kicking and screaming."

Two weeks later I was at a party and got talking to a bubbly, outgoing personality. It turned out he also was a funeral director but I found him the perfect party companion as he related some bizarre and astonishing stories. All in the best possible taste of course.

"Actually it was only yesterday," he told me, "that I was discussing headstones with a client. He'd been to a stonemasons and asked the price of a headstone. The relative thought it rather expensive. 'Oh, I know it sounds a lot,' said the stonemason, 'But once you've bought one, it lasts a lifetime."

Graham said a publican who had just passed away, requested that he should be placed in his coffin clutching a bottle of Jack Daniels. "But I think the strangest request we ever had was an elderly lady who had died leaving quite a lot of money and property and had requested specifically in her will that: "I be placed, face down in the coffin so I cannot see any of those hypocrites and vultures gathered around my grave."

"There is an unusual occurrence you might be interested in," said Graham. "We once had a lady who came to nearly all our funerals. She would masquerade as a distant relative and if anyone started to question her more closely, she would sniff loudly and dab feverishly at her eyes with a lace edged hankie. Anyone who was seen with the slightest trickle of tears or puffy eyes would get dabbed with the same lace hankie. She would even mingle with the real relatives patting their foreheads with a lavender scented, stick cologne - even the fellahs!"

He started to giggle, "I've just remembered a lady who had come to the Chapel of rest to see her husband. She was accompanied by her daughter, who had given us the clothes she wanted her father to be dressed in. They stood silently for some time, then the daughter decided to leave her mum on her own."

"I was feeling really choked," she told me, "but if I'd started to cry I thought it would upset Mum even more so I've come out here."

"After two or three minutes the mother joined her. I was surprised to see her looking so perky. She looked at her daughter and shaking her head said, 'your father will turn in his grave if he knew they'd put him in all those silly frilly things.'"

"The daughter explained that she'd chosen the things and she was sure her dad wouldn't mind."

"Mind? You have to be joking, he'd wouldn't be seen dead in things like that" and stormed out."

This time it was my turn to giggle.

My entertaining companion then told me a story which revolved around a widow who had told them that when her husband passed away, he'd been reading his favourite author Charles Dickens.

Graham told me: "She asked us to arrange to have a finger in the actual page he was reading when he died."

By now he was on a roll and we'd been ensconced in a dark corner, deep in conversation for over an hour and the other partygoers were getting increasingly curious as to what we could possibly be talking about. We heard rather disparaging remarks flying about but we ignored them all. This is what a reporter must feel like, hot on the trail of a good story.

"At one funeral," continued Graham, "One of the mourners had his arms around his sister's shoulders. She was extremely distressed, so he reached for the handkerchief nestling in his breast pocket and offered it to her. She was showered with confetti. He'd last worn the suit it at his wedding."

I was having difficulty getting it all down, as I wanted to be accurate, so made a mental note to try and learn shorthand as I was also in the process of writing four other books, all anecdotal. I apologised for my slowness. "That's okay," said Graham, "Anyway, I think that's about it, I really can't think of any more."

"No worries," I said, "You've been a star." and was just saying my grateful thanks when a fly started dive-bombing our corner with unerring accuracy for my nose.

"Oooh, just a minute," exclaimed Graham, "That's fly's reminded me of a time when we'd had really hot weather for days on end. As we were carrying the coffin into church I noticed that the pale cream roses on the top, seemed to be awash with expired bees. During the service I watched as a particularly dopey bee crawled unsteadily up a female's bare arm. The girl suddenly felt it, and started flapping at it hysterically, screaming very loudly as she did so. The whole congregation turned, wondering what had happened: Cries of: "What's wrong?" and "Oh, my God," filled the humid air. By then the poor creature had lazily joined its companions, collapsing in a comatose heap among the roses."

"I wouldn't mind," said Graham, "but the hymn they were about to sing was 'All Things Bright and Beautiful."

Suddenly we were aware of a figure looming over us. It was our hostess. "What are you two up to?" she asked, "You should both be mingling." The interruption was timed to perfection as Graham had come to an end of his story-telling, so I was able to put away my bulging notebook.

As I mingled I suddenly recalled a critique which had been given to Noel Coward's play, 'Sirocco.' It was described as "About as cheerful as a conference of undertakers, mainly because of the dreary dialogue."

I shall have to invite him to meet my friend Graham.

Most of the people I spoke to were male but I did meet one lady called Jacqueline, she told me that she'd gone to the local job centre and they put her on a training course to become a funeral director and the delights of embalming.

I suppose she could be justified in stating that the welfare state really does look after you - from the cradle to the grave.

On Radio Humberside's morning show a gentleman rang in to complain that a patient who had died was left in the ward all day.

"I hope they closed the curtains." said a shocked Peter Adamson.

"Oh yes they closed the curtains, but we all sat there knowing what was behind them."

Peter admitted it was a "rum do," and would try to find out what had happened from the hospital concerned.

There was a slight pause. "Oh, dear me," said Peter, "I've just noticed that the next record is Roy Orbison's, 'It's All Over,' we can't play that can we? Another very slight pause, "Oh, dear me, the one after that is , 'Stranger In Paradise,' which is nearly as bad. I know I'll turn the record over. Ah, that's better, Roy Orbison singing Blue Bayou."

Sighs of relief all round.

Louise was driving along the Clive Sullivan Way with her six-year old daughter Amanda, when suddenly the heavens opened and the windscreen wipers were having great difficulty in clearing the screen.

"Mummy?"

"Yes, darling?"

"Does it rain in heaven?"

Louise was stumped for a moment then answered, "I'm not really sure, I've never been there."

"Oh, that's all right, I'll ask Uncle Walter."

Her mother was curious. "Why do you think Uncle Walter will know?"

"Well he's got a computer and it tells him everything.

I was telling this story to a friend and she started to giggle. "You'll like the one about my granddad then," she said.

"Why, what happened?"

"Well his sister had just passed away and I had to go and tell him."

"I'm sorry Granddad, I said, but Auntie Hilda has just died. Granddad looked a bit downcast, then asked me. "How did you find out love, did she ring you?"

Peter G... said they were at the funeral of his mother. "She always looked on the black side of everything. In her eyes everything had a down side. On the day of her funeral, the weather was atrocious" Peter told me.

"It was bitterly cold and sheeting down with rain. Robin, my nine year old son attended the service. There was a pause in the proceedings and Robin piped up with, `Nana would be really happy if she knew it was such a rotten day wouldn't she?"

My friend Sheila told me about a farmer who had died and was laid out in the parlour of a small farmhouse. His three sons were paying their respects, when son number one said, "I've never seen Dad without his muffler. It doesn't look right somehow."

He went out, returning with a dark green scarf which he wrapped around his father's neck. "There, that was his favourite. He'll like that."

Son number two said, "That wasn't his favourite. He liked the blue one best." And proceeded to fetch it from the hall and wrapped that around the old man's neck.

Son number three, who had been quietly contemplating the proceedings, went out of the room, returning with a grey and white muffler, which without a word, he took off the other two and put his around their father's neck.

"Why have you done that?" asked his brothers..

"Because he always wore that on a special occasion and this is a special occasion."

They argued for some time, but eventually decided dad should be buried with all three mufflers.

My neighbour Mrs K... returned an invoice addressed to her recently departed father with the words: "Mr Williams deceased, new address not known." printed boldly across the page.

On one of my jaunts into foreign climes I saw a story in a local newspaper telling of a gentleman by the name of Michael Inat, who was somewhat surprised to receive a letter from the statistics department advising him: "According to our records, you died a year ago. Could you please confirm this."

Mr Inat wrote back confirming that he was not dead but that he was in fact alive and well. He told the reporter: "I couldn't resist asking the officials, 'why if you thought I was dead, did you bother writing to me in the first place?"

I also remember reading about the death of a member of parliament, it then went on to tell of an eager candidate who had rung and put himself foreward as a successor. "Sorry to hear of the recent death of Tom Atkins, " he said, "but is there any chance of me taking his place?" "Sure," replied the national agent, "If the undertaker has no objection."

Also spotted in a newspaper: "The deceased died at a local hospital after a long courageous battle with the doctors."

I was on holiday in California when I saw an undertakers called ' The Neptune Company.' Their blurb stated: "We consider ourselves a forward thinking company, so much so we are now considering offering our customers the option of having their loved one's remains blown up as part of a fireworks display. Ashes are launched from a barge in San Francisco Bay." It went on: "We are poised to take advantage of dramatic trends towards cremation as a simpler, dignified and more economic alternative to conventional burial."

That's what I call going out with a bang!

Another time during a flight to Majorca I was seated next to a sprightly 74 year old. We got chatting and she told me she'd been recently widowed and this was her first time abroad. "I'm really looking forward to it," she told me. Then leant down and picked up her flight bag. Out of it she produced a small brass urn. "My husband's in here." she said. I was just thinking how romantic when she carried on. "He was such a miserable bugger when he lived, I can't wait to show him what a good time I'm having now."

As they say, 'there's not a lot you can say to that.'


My husband Ray and I were discussing funerals. "I've no idea whether you prefer burial or cremation. It's very important. Just to put my mind at rest, what do you prefer?"

After a long deliberation Ray looked at me and said. "Surprise me!"

# GENERAL PRACTITIONERS

G.P's put up with an endless series of whining, whinging and complaining, so I thought I'd give them a chance to get their own back and asked a few doctors about comedic exploits with patients.

They of course could not mention names and I can't reveal the source of my information but if some of the stories are anything to go by they'd all make the grade as stand-up comedians.

"I had a patient who complained bitterly about the pills I'd prescribed," said Dr. K.... ."so I asked him what was wrong."

He explained: "I seem to be walking side-ways like a crab."

"So I said to him: I told you they had side-effects."

And then I met Dr J...

"A lady came in to see me and said she thought she had that fantasy flu what's going around."

"Fantasy flu?" I asked her.

"Yes, well I thought it was a bit like those fantasy pregnancies you get."

And what about the one from Dr. W...

"I had just syringed out Mr Clarke's ears and told him that one was a little inflamed so I would like him to keep an eye on it."

"That's going to be a bit difficult doc." he replied. "Will it be all right the wife does it?"

Joshua had to go to a doctor as his back was troubling him. He came home with some tablets the physician had prescribed to ease the nagging pain.

His wife also had been to the doctor's for trouble with her back..

"Wonder if he's given you the same as me."

"What sort's that then?" asked Joshua.

His wife went to get her bottle. "Well they're white ones."

"So's mine. What do they call 'em?"

"Uuumm! Ah, here we are. 'As before,' it says here."

"Mines different," said Joshua, "Mine says as directed"

And so it continued. I seemed to have tapped a comic reservoir.

While chatting to G.P.'s. I found that grateful patients are very fond of giving them something home-made, things like chutney and jam, even pressed flowers. One puzzled practitioner said he'd been given some dental fixative. "I don't even have false teeth," he told me. "But you name it, we have been offered it. We dont mind as long as it's not too expensive. I mean a Terry's Chocolate Orange will hardly affect our judgement will it?" He smiled and added, "Not unless I swallowed the thing whole!"

I asked what happened to unwanted gifts. "We have a Christmas lucky dip for all the office staff so it usually goes into that."

One Hull doctor had given a patient some ointment for piles. "He rang and asked for an urgent appointment. I saw him that afternoon. He came in clutching a small plastic bag. In it he'd placed a small purple lump which he'd passed when he'd gone to the loo. I looked at it carefully, then pressed it firmly, it split and squashed easily. They'd had fruit pie the night before and it was one of the pips." With a twinkle in his eye he said: "I suppose you could say he contracted Berry, Berry."

My friends three year old daughter, Tara was taken to the doctor with an upset stomach. When I asked her what the doctor had said to her, she replied: 'I've got a snail inside my tummy.' Mum laughed and said, "What he actually said was she had a tummy bug!"

In the bed next to me in hospital was Gladys, a lovely lady who'd had a knee replacement. She had been in hospital many times and was a keen observer of human nature so I was kept very busy recording her fascinating stories..

She told me she lived for a time in Bransholme, before the G.P's had a proper surgery and appointments were made at the Bodmin Road church. "I went to have a septic finger lanced, when he'd finished he realised he didn't have any dressings in the make-shift surgery, so he nipped out to the waiting room and asked the receptionist to pop to the nearest chemist to buy a box of elastoplast."

A husband went up to the receptionist to make an appointment on behalf of his pregnant wife, who needed an ante-natal check-up. He was asked: "How far is she?" To which he replied: "She's only up the road."

I think he felt rather embarrassed when she said: "No, I mean how many weeks pregnant is your wife?"

I was sitting in my doctor's surgery waiting my turn and doing what I do best, eavesdropping.

"I know somebody who changes her outfits twice a day." said a large 50 something, clad in purple jogging pants and an oversized yellow T-shirt.

"Never!" replied a twenty something, looking resplendent in a bright red anorak, green flowered skirt and blue trainers.

"Yes, and it's always bloody matching."

"Never."

"Mind you, my daughter-in-law only wears her clothes for a day."

"Never."

"Yes, and she comes from Glasgow."

"Bloody 'ell. They cut your throat if you go to Glasgow."

"Wonder if that's why she came to 'ull."

They say laughter is a wonderful tonic. I agree, that conversation perked me up no end.

Karl a practitioner in Hull said: "Recently I had an elderly lady in the surgery and I had to ask quite a few personal questions. Her answer to me was, 'I can talk about it, I can think about it, but I'm afraid I'm past doing it now.' Well she was 89."

An elderly patient asked Dr. G...if he'd ever had pills in those child proof bottles. He admitted he had.

"Can you open them?" she asked.

"With great difficulty" he told her.

"Well you're bloody clever then, 'cos I have to wait 'till my six year old grandson comes home to open them for me."

"Take these pills three times a day." Dr H.... told an elderly patient.

"How can I do that doctor?" she asked.

"If you forget what I've told you, it tells you on the side. I pointed to the bottle."

"Yes, I can see that, but if I take a pill three times a day, when I take it in the morning it'll be gone. Or do I just suck it for a bit?"

I couldn't argue with her logic, but she was deadly serious."

Do you smoke? More to the point have you ever tried to give up? Doctor's are often asked for magic remedies to help.

Dr K... told me: "One patient came to see me as her cough was really causing problems. I advised her to try nicotine pads to help her give up smoking. Put a new patch on every two days I told her. Three weeks later she returned. She made the most peculiar sound as she walked. I lifted her blouse to listen to her chest and found she had never taken off any of the patches. How she ever got washed I daren't think."

A doctor was visiting a patient who had been very depressed since the death of her husband.

"I couldn't get any satisfactory replies to my questions, so I tried another tack. What did your husband die of? I asked. She thought for a while then said brightly. 'He died of a Wednesday."

"I tried very hard not to laugh, so rooted around in my bag for a few minutes while I controlled myself. She was as right as rain within a week. All it took was a few kind words a dose of tonic pills."

I aked Dr T... if he had any strange or comic anecdotes. He shook his head. "Not that I can think of." Then gave a grin. "Well not so much comic as unusual," he said. "A nun came to see me." He paused. "I don't mean she was unusual but her problem was. She was suffering from a really stubborn rash on her scalp, which I couldn't identify. I eventually traced the reason. It was caused by the constant chafing of her wimple."

Dr Vernon Coleman - he writes a problem column in the Sunday People - said he was once talking to a patient when his chair broke and deposited him on the floor.

"I banged my nose and it bled. As I sat on the floor, the woman patient on the other side of the desk continued to tell me about her arthritis. She didn't pause to ask me if I was OK and didn't show the slightest concern."

# MATERNITY

Sign outside the Hedon Road Maternity Hospital
"Pick-up and drop. 15 minutes only"
Ooh, ladies if it was only that easy!

When I was in hospital having my son I was looked after by a nurse Day. Guess what her first name was? Bertha. She told me about a lady who had been in labour for over thirty hours.

"Her husband had been by her side for the last hour, as the baby's head was beginning to appear I yelled push, push. The husband thought I meant the baby and moved forward to push the babies head back."

At least it took my mind off my own labour, which was taking a tad too long in my opinion. But 18 hours later I was a proud mum.

The following day I was sat up in bed after the birth and the local vicar popped in to see me.

"Have you decided on a name?" he asked.

I smiled, thinking he would be impressed by our choice. "Adam," I replied.

"Ah," said the vicar. "Is that after Adam Faith the pop singer?"

Three months later, a friend remarked: "Aren't you lucky to have your figure back so quickly."

"Not really," I told her, "I was hoping to get someone else's."

Why, when you've been pushing and straining for what seems like a fortnight, do people take such pleasure in telling you about their Concorde-like delivery

One new mum told me she'd just had her fourth and it had popped out in minutes. "The first time," she said, "I didn't even realise I was pregnant. I was admitted to hospital with severe stomach cramps. While I was laid on a trolley waiting for the doctor to examine me, a young student nurse came to hold my hand. She went to the bottom of the trolley to re-arrange the sheet and as she lifted it up, saw a head appearing between my legs. I was giving birth. She rushed me into a nearby cubicle and delivered the baby. It was over in minutes. Suddenly the curtains were pulled aside and a doctor walked in to examine me. 'You're too late,' said the nurse, "She's just had a healthy six pound baby boy;" "I'd better go and tell the lady outside she's a grandma then", said the doctor. As he relayed the news, Mum's eyes opened in disbelief, she gave a sort of strangled gasp then crumpled in a heap at his feet. Another emergency, but not quite so exciting."

I was talking to Tony Richards an ambulance driver in Hull and he told me that while in the service he'd delivered fourteen babies, including a set of twins. He told me: "Even the mother didn't know she was expecting two and I had just turned away with one baby when she yelled that she was pushing again. Don't worry I told her, it'll be the afterbirth, but no, out popped another little head, screaming very loudly!"

This reminds me of a story a nurse told me: "A young mother was at the ante-natal clinic and the doctor told her she was expecting twins."

"Would you like to know the babies sex?" asked the doctor.

"No," she said, "I want to be surprised. Just tell me, are they the same?"

"No," replied the doctor.

But back to Tony Richards. "One week," he told me, "we'd been called out every night to deliver a baby, so on the sixth night (which was the last of our shift before a rest day) we were anxiously waiting for the jackpot, and were really disappointed when no baby needed our assistance into the world that night, although about a month later there were eight crews on duty and we delivered 19 babies between us. That must be some sort of record."

Gwen Laughton told me about the time she had to attend a maternity hospital.

"I was in my 60's and been diagnosed with cancer," she said, "I'd had chemotherapy and was on a drug which started up my periods. I was told to attend the maternity hospital in Cottingham and an ambulance came to pick me up. As we pulled up to the entrance the driver asked me if I was sure I'd got the right place. You should have seen all those young, mum's-to-be faces when this grey haired granny came and plonked herself among them. But that's where the gynaecology department was, so that's where I had to go."

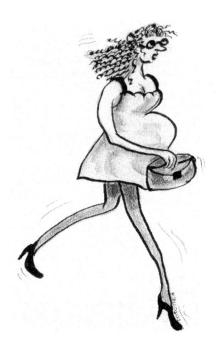

A maintenance engineer was required in a supervisory capacity at the Townend Maternity Home. The advert read: "Maintenance engineer required. Must have experience of dealing with labour."

Perfect job then.

Gladys Whitaker said she was hospitalised for the duration of her pregnancy and she was in a side ward, except this room was also used for radiation treatment.

"Whenever the equipment needed to be used they would wheel me out into the main ward until they'd finished and then wheel me back again. We are talking 1960's here and thankfully things have changed a bit since then."

"I'd had two miscarriages, so special precautions had to be taken during intercourse, as the sperm was having difficulty making their way up my tubes, I was advised to regularly take my temperature and when it hit the desired total we had to make love. But there was a problem. My rear end had to be up in the air. Doctors suggested I propped myself up on pillows, so the sperm could have an easier passage.

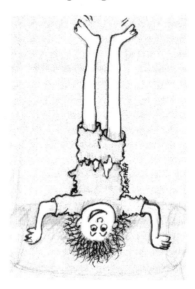

First I'd yell for my husband and we were so determined those sperm were going to make it, I ended up just about standing on my head. Wow!" said Gladys, "Did we have some fun trying to make a baby."

"Did it work?" I asked.

"Certainly did. We had a beautiful son."

A nurse in Hedon Road maternity hospital was telling an auxiliary she'd just delivered a baby to a 55 year old woman. "It was her twelfth," she said.

"Bloody 'ell," replied her colleague. "She's a glutton for punishment. If it'd been me, I'd have sewn it up by now."

A patient nearby overheard and told them. "Oh, that's not an option. They do it for the money you know. The more kids, the more money they get. Scandalous if you ask me."

She paused, looked puzzled, then asked: "Can you have it sewn up?"

Nurse Roberts told me she had been talking to the grandmother of a young patient.

"She was only sixteen and the grandmother was convinced it had all been a terrible mistake. 'Something's wrong,' she told me, 'because to have a baby you have to consume first and I'm certain our Tracy never has."

A girl was being shown how to bath her baby and given tips on general care.

"Any questions?" asked the nurse.

"Just one thing you haven't mentioned," replied the young mum. "What time should I wake a new baby in the mornings?"

I giggled at this remark but the nurse soon put me in my place. "You need scoff," she said, "But I had one lady who was really worried that her baby might arrive while she was asleep."

Brenda, a doctor in a large practice, was discussing hysterectomy with a patient.

"How many children have you got?" she asked.

"Nine. Eight boys and a girl."

"Were you disappointed," asked the doctor. She was going to continue with, 'having so many boys,' but the patient interrupted.

"I bloody was. Who wants a girl when you've so many boys?"

Brenda said she was surprised at the answer, but the patient went on to explain.

"I had to buy new clothes didn't I? And as for the sleeping arrangements. A bloody nightmare, that's what it is. A bloody nightmare."

Actually that story reminds me of the time I had just returned home after giving birth.

I was sat in a chair with my son, when the window cleaner arrived. He knocked on the window and mouthed "What did you get?"

"A boy." I replied.

He nodded and carried on with his work. When he came to the door for his money, he asked,

"How about swopping for twin girls?"

"Not at the moment. But I'll keep it in mind. Why do you ask?"

"I've got seven girls and that includes three sets of twins. We tried three times and every time it was twins and all girls. We decided we would try one more time for a boy. The wife had a test, so early on we knew there was only one baby and it was another girl, so we decided to call it a day."

I couldn't resist commenting: "What a funny name."

# MEDICAL RECORDS

A doctor who shall be nameless passed on some interesting entries from patients records.

"I must admit to one that I was guilty of, but realising what I'd put, changed it. I'd first written, 'The patient has been depressed since seeing me.' It's so easy to do and when you're very busy you seldom read the entry back."

He said one of his favourites was: "The patient has not been known to commit suicide before."

I couldn't decide which was my favourite so I'll let you choose.

"She's numb from her toes down."

"She has two teenage children but no other abnormalities."

"She is to refrain from sexual intercourse until next I see her in my office.'

"Since the patient stopped smoking his smell is returning.'

"Sinuses run in the family.'

"The surgeon is looking at Mrs Grafton's leg on Thursday and we'll take it from there."

# MEDICAL SCHOOL

An intern was examining a 30 year old woman. She had been admitted with stomach pains. He commented on her hysterectomy and appendectomy scars but was puzzled by a third scar down the centre of her stomach. He had to ask the patient what it was for. The lady peered to see where he was pointing and burst out laughing and told him: "That's the mark from the seam of my tights."

A young house doctor told me about the time he was still attending medical school: "I had to collect my urine for twenty-four hours, so I could check my kidneys were in working order. Obviously I started with my first pee of the day and took the bottle with me to college for the top ups. That night about six of us went to a nearby pub, which we knew was frequented by a few tasty single girls. I was busy chatting up a particularly spicy blonde when my so called friends added some beer and whisky to my urine sample. And it had to happen didn't it? I was stopped by the police on my way home. I was convinced I had nothing to worry about but I was a borderline case so they asked me to go to the station to give a sample. Thinking I'd save time, I poured some of the urine from my bottle into their receptacle. Oh, boy, it showed nearly pure alcohol content. It took some explaining I can tell you. I insisted on a blood test and it proved I was telling the truth."

The same student remembered the time they all went out to celebrate the end of exams: "Twenty of us decided we'd live it up and go for a meal. None went overboard with the menu but when the bill arrived we could only muster .37p between us for the tip. We all made a quick exit feeling very guilty as the waitress had been really helpful."

# MISCELLANEOUS

I'm at a loss to categorise some of the bizarre events I've witnessed. For instance take the tale of Mrs Williamson. She'd been admitted as an emergency late on the Sunday night. Her son came to visit the following morning and was dumbfounded as he watched staff rushing around like "headless chickens" as he put it. There were nurses, doctors, porters and domestic staff all trying to get their work done around commodes which were being expertly weaved around patients who plodded around with their zimmer frames in attack mode, and buzzers were being pressed from every which way but loose. He asked me if this was normal and I told him "very."

"Right," he said, "I'm going to sort this out." and strode out of the ward to the nurses station beyond.

For the next five days until she was discharged, his mum received gold star treatment. I was intrigued, to say the least at this miraculous turn-around. Was she somebody famous? The son revealed all. "Never fails," he told me. "I gave the sister on duty fifty pounds to look after my mother's every need."

I tackled the sister and she denied it. "We have a code governing what we can and can't accept from patients and cash is a definite no, no." She smiled, then added, "But of course you can make a donation to the ward if you so wish."

Problem solved!

My friend Ray Scott had suffered a heart attack and was

prescribed daily exercise, so he thought it would be a good idea to join a walking club, thinking that would improve his fitness.

He rang me and mentioned he'd been "Hell walking."

"Don't you mean hill walking?" I asked.

"You might call it hill walking, I call it Hell walking. I'm not going any more."

"But you have to take some sort of excersise," I told him.

"But I do," he said, "I walk regularly."

"Where?"

"I never use the bapper to change channels, I always walk briskly to and from the set. Sometimes as often as six times a night." he said mischievously.

Mrs Boland said she'd just collected some tablets for the dog and put them next to her own on the table: "My husband came in and told me I'd have to be careful as we didn't want any accidents. I was really touched by this, " she told me, "Until he continued, "those dog tablets cost a lot of money so are too expensive to waste."

A young patient was admitted for a tonsillectomy operation. Her mother was a constant visitor. A few days later, Chloe was soon back to her chatty self. She told her mother that: "A man put a funny prickle in my arm then I disappeared."

Countdown was being shown on the television and patients were asked if they wanted to watch it.

"Oh, yes," remarked one girl, her arms stuck out at right angles in a huge brace. "I always do it with them."

"I do as well." commented a sixty year old, for whom the years had not been kind. She continued. "I can do all the words but my figures bloody awful."

Nick a passing male nurse, ever ready with a quip said. "You can say that again Joan."

She took it in good faith but was heard to mutter, "Cheeky bugger."

I was in a side ward, feeling a bit sorry for myself, a blood transfusion had just been actioned, but at least the automatic morphine drip, inserted in my back was keeping the pain at bay. From the nurses station I could hear ribald laughter. It went on for some time. What was happening? I rang my buzzer.

A head popped round the door. "Why all the merriment?" I asked. "I hate lying here and listening to you enjoying yourselves. Can't you all come in here and share it with me? I need a good laugh."

"I'll be back in five minutes to explain," said Mandy. True to her word she returned to tell the tale.

Evidently when Mandy was in her late teens she started 'courting' a trainee psychiatrist and he used to practise his skills on her.

"I was trying one out on the other nurses," she said and explained.

"First you have to imagine you are going along a path, any path, you must choose what it's like, stony, grassy, meandering, straight, it's your choice. Okay?" I nodded. "On the path you see a key on the ground and you pick it up. Look at it and decide whether it's heavy, small, gold, rusty, you decide again. Then go through a wood, how dense or overhung it is, again, your decision. At the edge of the wood is some water. Is it stagnant, fresh, running fast? Again you decide. Lastly at the far side of the water you see a wall, high enough to hide the view on the other side. What sort of wall is it? Do you want to climb over to see what's at the other side?"

I had all these images in my mind when Mandy asked me to describe what I'd 'seen'

My path was a grassy track, through fields of wild flowers. I was told "That's your path through life. What about the key?"

"Oh, that was large, old and very ornate."

"That shows your view of wealth and possessions. Now before you describe the water, would you like to swim in it?" asked Mandy.

"Definitely," I told her, "I can't wait to try it out."

She laughed and told me: "The water is considered your view of sex." Ah, all was revealed. That's what was causing all the merriment. Mandy said, "Some just wanted to test it with a toe first, some didn't want to go in at any price and one said she'd throw off all her clothes and plunge in head first." By now you'd almost forgotten about the wall, but evidently that is your view of the future. Are you the type to take risks or do you prefer to stay on familiar ground.

Try it on your friends. I guarantee it's great fun and livens up a party no end.

A manager came into the ward and I heard him ask the sister: "Anything you want?"

"Yes," she replied, "Some wood and nails."

"Wood and nails?"

"Yes. I'd like to knock up a few extra beds."

Anne Waddingham said she'd been rushed into hospital while she was on holiday in Cyprus.

"I only had a smattering of the language but never-the-less made friends with one of the nurses. When I was released she invited me to her home. She was very insistent, so a few days later I went along to see her."

"I've been in hospital many times," said Anne, "But I have to admit, it's the very first time a nurse has asked me home for tea."

Gwen Laughton was in hospital with a broken femur after an accident. This entailed her whole body being encased in a plaster cast. She told me: "All my friends brought me knitting needles to push down the plaster cast and relieve the tickling which desperately needed a scratch. They eventually stopped bringing them. I lost five in the bowels of the cast!"

Karen said they'd admitted a young man who'd been in a motor-cycle accident. He had a broken arm, leg and several smashed teeth. The nurse told me: "In the next bed was George who had been admitted with a compound fracture of his tibia and I heard him ask the young man how he'd got injured. When he explained about the accident, George told him he'd given up riding a motor-bike as it was too dangerous. I burst out laughing," said Karen, because I knew how George had come to be so badly injured."

I couldn't resist asking: "How?"

"Skydiving! and he was 69!"

A farmer's wife from the village of Swine, had been admitted as an emergency to the hospital. Her husband visited later that day. He was taken into a small room and told to wait for a few minutes. The nurse told him they'd had to operate on his wife and everything had gone well, but he was asked to wait as the doctor would like a word. Soon the door opened and a young female doctor came in, still clad in the green operating gown and cap, complete with wellies.

They chatted for a few minutes with the doctor explaining the problem and told him he could now visit his wife on the ward.

"Thanks, that's reet nice of you," said the farmer, then with a gleam in his eye asked, "Are you married?"

The doctor nodded.

"Bloody good job," said the farmer, "'cos you look a right bugger in that outfit, tha's less dress sense than me."

I asked a nurse what the worst injuries she'd ever seen.

"I've been a nurse for twenty years," she said, "but easily the worst I ever saw was a lady who had been riding a donkey on Scarborough sands, her foot had slipped in the stirrup and it had shot up her leg, causing horrific injuries to her fufu."

A staff nurse on Ward 70, told me about the lady who had to be admitted during school holidays so she left her son with her mother.

"The boy visited his mum every day at 1.30 and went at 3.30pm, always on his own. We found out that grandma went to bingo every day and there was no-one to look after him, so she would put him on a bus to the hospital, then he'd have to find his own way back. He was seven years old."

Stella in a nearby bed was telling an auxiliary about her grandson. "He's got a new car you know and he desperately wanted a steering wheel cover to fit it." Mmm, I thought, that's a strange shape for a car, but I digress. She continued: "He was coming to visit me and he had three hours to spare but his mum had to come without him. She'd left him at home trying to stitch the thing on." I fantasised again. What part of his anatomy would it fit? The voice carried on: "He'd already broken three needles. He can't get them through the leather. My Julie left him at home swearing a lot but she says he's determined to have a nice cover on his steering wheel. He was supposed to be bringing them but they've had to come on the bus."
"Why, can't he drive without one?" asked Janet.
"Ooh, he likes to do things proper."
"Maybe he should have bought a fluffy one."
"Ooh, 'e couldn't do that. 'e's a fellah and fellah's don't 'ave fluffy ones."
She'd obviously led a very sheltered life!

A patient was trying to have a crafty smoke under his bedclothes. A nurse ran over to his bed and pointed to all the signs, "NO SMOKING" and explained that apart from everything else, there were cylinders of oxygen in the ward. "Now," she said sternly." "If you'd caused an explosion and I'd have been killed. I'd have come back and haunted you for ever more."

Gladys Whitaker was woken up in the middle of the night thinking she was being strangled. "It was only the young girl in the next bed, who decided she was feeling lonely and wanted to give me a cuddle, except she had her arms around my neck. Luckily a nurse had seen what was happening and extricated me just in time."

Gloria gave a diabetes patient a little stick, a clinistic, to check his urine. "Go and pee on this," she told him. "If diabetes is present the blue patch on the stick turns brown." When he returned the indicators were shrivelled away. "Bloody 'ell," said the nurse, "What have you been drinking?" "Well I was trying to snatch a crafty smoke and dropped my ciggie on it."

The next test showed he was clear, but he got a roasting for the cigarette escapade.

Wendy, always sat on her bed with one leg tucked underneath and the other dangling over the side. Bethany, a small, blonde, five year old, was watching her with fascination. Suddenly she asked: "Mummy, did the doctors take that lady's leg off?"

I was having an afternoon nap. Suddenly I'm aware of someone shaking my arm and calling my name.

"Dorothea, I've a pill for you. Now don't wake up quickly or you'll give yourself a headache."

Thanks a bunch!

A very overweight lady was admitted and in the evening her family came to visit.

When they'd gone, she asked me if I'd noticed her daughters. "Yes," I said, "You must be very proud of them. They're both very pretty." I didn't add that they were also at least two stone overweight. So the next question floored me.

"Do you think they're fat?"

I hesitated, I had no idea what answer she expected and I'm not one to hurt anyone's feelings, so was humming and hawing a bit when she indignantly told me the fourteen year old was slimming. "Slimming! At her age. I ask you. She's the perfect weight for her size. But she wont listen to me or her dad. I despair I really do."

I nodded sympathetically but said nothing as I'd also noted Dad, who can't have been more than 5'8, weighed at least fifteen stone. As they say beauty is in the eye of the beholder.

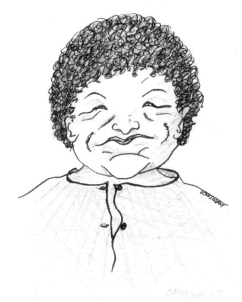

"Have you ever met Dr. B...?" asked a nurse.

"Yes," I admitted, "But only briefly."

"Did you understand anything he said?" she asked.

"Well he did go on a bit," I said.   "Go   on   a   bit!"   she exclaimed, "I swear the man's had a clarity by-pass operation."

Gill had taken her three-year-old grand-daughter to see an elderly neighbour, who had been confined to bed for a few days. The bedroom was delightfully decorated in pale blue, even the sheets and pillowcases were blue and to top it all Mrs Richardson was clad in a fetching blue nightie. Phillipa was unusually quiet and nothing could persuade her to say a word to Grandma's friend. As they were walking back to the car, Phillipa asked: "Nan, why was that lady sitting in the sky? Was it Heaven?"

I worked for several years for a market research company and met some fascinating characters on my travels. In fact I've just completed a book about them, with a selection of cartoons, for as they say, 'seeing is believing - Anyway I was doing an interview on healthy living and talking to a 72 year old.

He drew a sharp intake of breath when I told him the subject.

"Waste of time love," he told me. "At my age everything either leaks, wilts or it's fallen off."

While in my car listening to the local radio station. An elderly lady was discussing the operation she'd just had for cataracts.

"I was fully conscious throughout," she told Ian Hunter, the presenter.

Ian added that he thought the patient was exceptionally brave. "I can't ever see me being conscious if they had to operate on my eyes."

I liked the 'see me' remark, but it got better as later I heard him announce: "This is Radio Humberside on 88.8 FM and here is the three o'clock news." The newscaster began: "The government today face a knife-edge vote today in parliament."

Ouch!

Sylvia Giles recalls the time she was assisting a doctor in giving a patient a lumbar puncture.

"He didn't seem to mind at all," said Sylvia, "When suddenly he lunged forward and clamped his teeth into my thigh. I retained a beautiful set of teeth imprints on my thigh for weeks and I don't think my husband Barrie, ever really believed me"

Gwen Laughton was a wonderful chirpy character who had come to Hull in the eighties, having spent most of her life in Margate and Southend. She still had an evocative accent and constantly regaled me with a multitude of memories from her childhood, her courting days and wartime England.

When she was eleven she was diagnosed as having T.B. In those days the only known cure was a years bed rest, she told me: "When they brought the screens round for you to go to the loo, I would take the opportunity for some exercise and jump up and down on the bed. Problem was my head could be seen bobbing up and down behind the screen and a nurse would come and stop me."

"The young girl in the bed next to me had been told she had to have a tonsillectomy but she died on the operating table. Mum and Dad came to see me a few days later and said that the doctor thought I should also have my tonsils out. This scared the living daylights out of me, so the next night, about eleven o'clock, I did a runner. A policeman stopped me and asked what I was doing out at that time of night. I fibbed and told him I'd been to a friends. When I got home my parents were furious and Mum rang the hospital to come and take me back. They put me under house arrest. My bed was wheeled into a little side room where I was confined and just to make sure I couldn't get out, they pushed a cabinet in front of the door. Nobody could hear me if I wanted anything. Can you believe that a sick eleven year old would be locked away in solitary like that?."

"The hospital was right on the front at Margate and some German boats shelled the coastline, smashing all our windows. They never replaced them. They said we needed fresh air anyway, so we all suffered."

"But it wasn't all bad, while I was there, King George VI, had arranged for some tropical fruits to be distributed to hospitals. You should have seen what they sent. We'd never seen anything like it in our lives. Everybody hated the watermelons, but I loved them. I thought they were great and ate them every day for a week." Gwen also recalled when she was a patient in a hospital in the 50's.

"At night, she told me, "the drinks trolley would make it's way very slowly round the ward."

"Why slowly? I asked.

"Ah, because these were drinks with a difference. They were the real thing. Whisky, brandy, sherry, in short, anything you fancied. I was an innocent sixteen year old, but I was persuaded to try a milk stout as I'd been diagnosed anaemic. I loved it," she told me, "In fact I've drunk it ever since."

I was fascinated by this story and asked how much the patients were charged for their nightly tipple. "Nothing," she said, "It was all free."

Like Gwen I was also a patient in hospital in the 50's, during the time of the polio outbreak, I was rushed to Beverley Westwood Hospital on suspicion of contracting the dreaded disease, but it turned out nothing more sinister than pneumonia. I normally sleep without any pillows so found it more than a tad difficult to find the arms of Morpheaus sitting upright. I'd just persuaded myself that sitting up to sleep was cool, when I was paid a visit by the doctor. There he stood at the end of my bed, a round, genial man, with wispy white hair curling in tendrils around his ears. Very fetching. Anyway he announced I was to have a lumbar puncture and that would entail lying flat with my feet higher than my head. Oh, crikey, here we go again!

While chatting to Gwen, a patient nearby was refusing to have a bath. She was getting very irate. We heard her shout: "I thought they'd done away with them things years ago." What could she mean? The nurses were also intrigued and asked her what on earth she was taking about. All was revealed. She had been told a hoist would have to be used to get her into the bath. She screamed at them: "They dunked witches in them things in the olden days."

All was explained and a pacified patient went quietly!

Allan Rowlands, a nurse at a local hospital, said he was negotiating a wheelchair down a ramp leading from the main entrance: "Suddenly both grips came off the handle of the wheelchair and it started to career down the slope while I was left standing there, firmly grasping two rubber grips. The terrified patient was really panicking, so I ran like a maniac and just managed to grab it before it catapulted into the shrubbery. I don't know who was the most shocked, the patient or me."

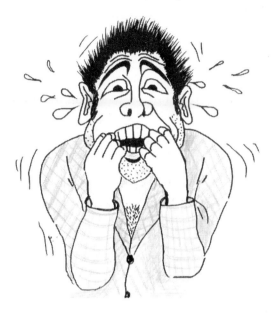

"It must have been something in the air," said Allan, "because about an hour later two technicians were manhandling a huge x-ray machine, which were used in the 60's, down the same slope. Suddenly they lost control and it developed a life of its own, heading towards a lone doctor trudging upwards. He stood firm, holding out his arms like a father waiting to clasp a child to the paternal breast. Not a good idea, he ended up flattened underneath the thing, suffering a broken arm and a few bruised ribs, but guess what? They had to use that machine to check his injuries!"

Allan also recalled the time when he was working in a hospital with an extremely wide corridor. "Wards were all along one side and administration offices on the other. It was Christmas and we'd been celebrating with the patients. Suddenly the junior doctors decided, it would cheer everyone up if they decorated a mini with garlands and tinsel and drive it down the corridor. The car was suitably attired, the driver got in, revved the engine to huge cheers and headed for the entrance, except their calculations were slightly adrift. It stuck in the doorway. They did manage to get it out without too much damage, but they were right about cheering everyone up. It worked a treat."

As Allan turned away the bell signalling the end of visiting was sounded. I heard Bettina in the next bed call her boy-friend back. "I forgot to ask you," she said, "But could you bring some hygiene pads in tomorrow?"

He looked a little perplexed but said nothing and went on his way. The next night he returned and gave Bettina a small paper bag. She opened it up and inside found three brillo pads!

A Saudi Arabian businessman needed a special blood replacement and it could only be done at one specialised hospital in England. The consultant rang the hospital concerned and they advised they only had six private beds and they were full, but they did have a space on the NHS general ward. The Saudi was not impressed but offered to give the hospital nearly a quarter of a million pounds if they could treat him in a private room. "Sorry, it doesn't make the slightest difference," said a hospital spokesman. "We haven't a private bed."

"Even for quarter of a million?" asked a dumfounded consultant.

"Even for half-a-million." he was told.

They found out that a consultant in America could carry out the procedure, so the Saudi businessman travelled over for the treatment and made a full recovery. The States were more than happy to accommodate their wealthy patient.

I'm sure there is a moral there somewhere, can any of you tell me what it is?

A nurse told me about a lady celebrating her 100th birthday. She was extremely fit and able for her age.

The local press went to the Nursing Home to interview her and take photographs.

"Is there anything you can't do?" asked the reporter.

"There is," Rose said emphatically.

The reporter, pencil poised, "And what's that?" he asked.

"Die, that's what I can't do. Die!"

It was June '99 and we'd had thunderstorms all day, but at night they became ferocious. We were all sitting bolt upright as the storm raged outside. First, all the lights went off, not a great problem as the whole ward was illuminated with the sheet lightening, while the thunder crashed and rolled about the heavens. Then the automatic doors stayed firmly shut. While the electrics were being sorted out we sprang a leak in the roof just outside the toilets, so nurses were hard pressed to attend to patients needs in the intermittent light, as well as mop up the deluge, which was increasing by the minute. Workmen had to be called out as several wards had been overcome by the elements. We thought we had problems but we found out later that ward one had rain pouring in so hard they'd had to evacuate everyone to nearby corridors.

Nobody got much sleep that night in Cottingham.

# NIGHTS

When I'm first admitted to hospital, as most patients, I find it difficult to sleep. But in the eighties, wards were much larger and noisier, not partitioned off into smaller units as they are today. You could see everything, as of course could the nurses. It was my third night, about half-past two in the morning, when sister popped her head around the door and asked staff nurse to help out in a near-by ward as they had an emergency, leaving a young nurse, freshly out of nursing school, on her own.

"Don`t worry," sister told her, "If anyone rings it'll only be for a bedpan."

Staff had been gone for about ten minutes when a buzzer went. She tiptoed down the ward past snoring patients and saw an elderly lady gesticulating wildly.

She quietly went to the bedside.

"Do you want a bedpan Mrs Wilson?"

"No, I don't," answered the old lady. "You've got to do something."

She sounded quite agitated. "There's somebody in bed with me."

"You're imagining it Mrs Wilson." said Gloria, and started to re-arrange the pillows.

"I know what's what and there's somebody in here with me."

The young nurse suddenly remembered someone telling her, all hospitals had ghosts. She gulped and looked around nervously, still trying to re-assure Mrs Wilson.

"Look, I know you think I'm a dotty old woman, but there's somebody in my bed I tell you and they've just bitten my bottom."

She looked earnestly into the face of the wide eyed girl and continued. "My husband used to do that when we were courting, I bet it's 'im, so can you tell 'im to stop it. I can't do with it at my age."

By now Gloria was shivering with fright, so making her excuses, returned to her desk. She wasn't quite sure what she should do.

The buzzer sounded again and she stood up holding tightly onto the edge of the small table for support. She felt quite faint. `Oh, God,` she thought. `What shall I do?"

But the cavalry was at hand. Staff came striding through the swing doors. Gloria nearly hugged her with relief.

Patting her gently on the arm, she said. "Come on, I'll show you its only an old woman's imagination. Probably the sheets have creased up and they feel funny."

They set off in the old ladies direction. Gloria walked nervously behind.

They stood at each side of the bed. Mrs Wilson repeated her story.

Staff gave her an enigmatic smile and proceeded to strip off the top sheet and straighten the bottom one.

"Just turn to your right Mrs Wilson, so I can pull the bottom sheet across."

The patient did as she was told and as she did so a set of false teeth which had been clamped into her rear-end for the last half-hour, fell onto the bedding.

Oh well, another ghost story hits the dust.

The following night the nurse had to wake a patient to take a pill. She gently shook her shoulder to rouse her. The patient stirred and asked what was the matter. Nurse explained. "Pills, bloody pills." shouted the patient, . "You mean you've woken me up in the middle of the bloody night ( it was 10.15pm ) to take a bloody pill. I've been in here for three days and this is the first time I've managed to get to sleep and you spoil it." The tirade continued unabated. She refused to listen to the importance of the medication and dragging her clothes out of the locker started to get dressed. Sister was called for, but she couldn't pacify her either. The patient insisted they ring her husband to come and take her home and plonked herself on the bed, resplendent in fur coat and ski boots. About forty minutes later hubby appeared. He sat on the bed and cuddled her. It became so amorous we asked the nurse to draw the curtains. They were ensconced behind them for over an hour. Suddenly the curtains opened, he walked out with a wide grin and announced: "She's all right now, I've tucked her up and you wont hear another peep out of her. Just give me a ring any time you have any trouble with her, I'll soon sort it," and with that strode out of the ward giving everyone a cheery wave on his way.

Now that's what I call a bedside manner! But she still hadn't taken her pill.

I soon learnt to ignore all the extraneous noises and fall into a deep sleep, but after I'd been a patient for about three months, for some reason my body refused to relax and succumb to Morpheous. It continued for three weeks. My eyes were red rimmed, sore and filled with sand - well it certainly felt like that! Pills just gave me a raging headache. In the previous weeks I had contracted pneumonia and pleurisy.

In fact I had become so ill, I was 'barrier nursed' for two weeks. This means the patient is isolated and staff and visitors have to wear masks and gowns at all times. The same cups, saucers and cutlery have to be used and only immediate family are allowed to visit. My twenty year old son was not amused when he was ordered to don a fetching green gown, mask and hat before entering my domain. The sight of my two favourite fellahs looking like escapees from ER was an instant pick-me-up.

But back to the sleeping, as I was in a side ward they would leave the television permanently on. The medical staff hoped it would have a soporific effect on me.

I never thought I would be pleased to be bedbound and in solitary confinement with only the television for company, but there's always a silver lining if you look hard enough. This was Olympic year and I am an athletics nut. There was an adulteration of sport for hours on end. I watched re-runs of the re-runs. Two in the morning or two in the afternoon it was all the same to me. I won't say I enjoyed my incarceration but by golly it improved my spirits no end.

My insomnia did have another redeeming feature. It made me privy to some very unusual happenings.

I remember one particular night, it would be about 1.00am, when I saw a patient go down to the end of the ward and have a word with the nurses. I heard her tell them: "Somebody has just tried to get into bed with me."

"You must have been dreaming," said staff nurse, "We've been sat by the door all night and no-one has come in."

"You can say what you like," said Sarah, "but somebody tried to get into bed with me."

"Let's go and have a look," said the nurse. The patients bed was checked and as they thought, it was empty. The patient was adamant and insisted the lights were put on. Most were awake by now anyway, so the nurses agreed. Not a strange body in the patients bed, but they did find an extra empty bed! They walked slowly up the ward to see if there was two in a bed somewhere. Nothing. Then a patient said, "What's that under Sarah's bed?" This was the lady who'd complained of an intruder, and there sure enough just peeping out from the end of her bed, were a pair of white bed socks.

The body attached to the socks steadfastly refused to come out and insisted on seeing a doctor, but she wouldn't say why. All the ward was now alert and expectant. After half-an-hour they admitted defeat and called the doctor.

About twenty minutes later, in walked the young house doctor, but she still refused to come out from under the bed, so the doctor crawled under the bed to talk to her. Ten minutes later he crawled out followed by the patient. She quite happily climbed back into her bed and within minutes was fast asleep.

The problem? Well there were two actually. She first complained about the chatting which went on in the ward and had insisted being moved to a, "Yak-free zone."

Then went on to tell the doctor, the nurse on dinner duty wouldn't give her the treacle pudding she'd wanted. The patient was diabetic!

Another night, this time about 3.00am, I heard the lady opposite my door, buzz for the nurse.

"What's wrong Clara?"

"I've wet the bed."

"Oh, God not again. I told you if you do it again you'll have to sleep in it."

"If I do, will I get king kof in my bum?"

"Very likely."

"It's all right for you nurses." said Clara. "When you get to my age you never know if you'll wake up or not."

"Rubbish! It's too bloody hot to get buried in the cemetery in this weather."

"Don't tell me about hot. My legs are burning up. I've got the wrong bandages on."

"They're the same bandages as you always have Clara."

"No, they're not. Nurse told me they're six, not three."

"Yes that's right. Six inches wide. So they'll be better as they don't overlap so much."

"No, you're wrong. There's twice as many bandages as normal. You're always getting things wrong. You make them worse."

"But Clara, the doctor's told you they're much better."

"You're wrong. I'm telling doctor about you."

"Good, you do that. Now do you want changing or not?"

"Not by you, thank you very much. I'll wait."

"Please yourself." She started to walk away. But Clara hadn't finished.

"By the way, you never brought me any water for my teeth."

"I did, but you were asleep and I couldn't see them on your locker."

"You bloody wouldn't would you? I've still got them in."

"No wonder I couldn't find them then."

"Well why didn't you take them out?"

"You wouldn't have been very happy if I'd woken you rooting about in your mouth would you?"

"You seem to be happy rooting about everywhere else. So why stop at my mouth?"

"Look we're keeping everyone awake. Go back to sleep I've got other patients to see."

"Bet their bloody legs aren't hot."

Clara eventually went to sleep and didn't stir until gone eight o'clock. I hate to think what the smell was like.

I awoke at just after midnight to find a pink shrouded figure with a silver halo of hair busying itself around my locker. I soon realised it was ninety-two year old Violet who'd been admitted from an old peoples home with acute breathing problems, but she had improved considerably and had decided it was time to do some housework and as I was nearest the door, it was my bedside table which was getting the treatment. I pressed the buzzer and a nurse soon led her gently away, telling her it all looked wonderful and what a good girl she'd been.

It happened on another three occasions. I had the cleanest locker in the hospital. Well nearly, she was dusting them down with her knickers!

"I consider myself one of the luckiest people in this hospital." Sarah told a nurse.

"Why?"

"Because I've spent five days in this ward with seven other patients and not one snores."

I know how she feels.

But in a nearby ward, it was the exact opposite, nearly everyone snored. It got so bad that in sheer desperation one patient decided to go and sleep on a chair in the day room. A nurse watched her then went to investigate.

"Doesn't it drive you mad with all those people snoring away?" asked the patient.

Smiling the nurse replied: "No, it's people like you who can't sleep, who drive us mad.

# NURSING HOMES

Minden told me about the time she was on night duty at Ferriby Hall, an old people's home outside Hull. "I was walking up some stairs late at night and came across a young boy with a lace collar. He disappeared around a corner. I ran after him but couldn't find anything. I was a bit concerned as children were not allowed in the home, but after searching all the open areas had to concede defeat. The next morning the gardener popped in and I mentioned it to him."

"I must be getting old," I told him, "but I would have sworn I saw something."

"The gardener burst out laughing. "You mean no-one's told you about our ghost?"

"Ghost. What ghost? I asked him. "Well it's two actually," he told me, "A young boy, who's usually accompanied by a lady in a crinoline. But not to worry, I'm told they're always smiling." I couldn't believe it. You mean I actually saw a real ghost. This amused the gardener who told me he wasn't sure about the 'real' bit, but it was definitely a ghost I'd seen. It's a bit scary really, " said Minden, "he looked so real. She pondered for a moment. "It's a shame but I never saw him again."

In the same home Minden recalls the time she heard a noise coming from a married couple's room. They were 91 and 87 and had been married over 45 years.

"I was a bit concerned one might be ill, so went to investigate. I listened outside the door for a minute and from what I heard I was convinced they were up to nookie, but as they were both rather frail and arthritic, I thought I'd better make sure."

"I peeped around the door and to my amazement saw the woman straddling the old man. She was heaving up and down, shouting loudly at her husband with each bounce. Rather startled I was going to withdraw when I realised what she was saying and they were definitely not having fun. She was yelling: "My mother said I shouldn't have married you, and with each word was pressing a pillow over his face trying to smother him. I managed to pull her off, while her nonagenarian husband kept muttering: "The woman's mad, completely mad.""

"We put her in a separate room until she calmed down."

"Any idea what started it off?" I asked.

"No, hadn't a clue and neither would spill the beans, but they asked to be reunited the next day and we never heard another peep out of them."

"The following night was Christmas Eve and we were looking forward to being entertained by a group of carollers. Matron approached a resident who had refused to have a bath or have her hair washed for over three weeks, and said to her:

"Millie, it would be nice if you have a bath and hair-do before the carollers come wouldn't it?"

"No, it wouldn't," answered Millie. "It's too cold."

"But the bathroom's heated and it would be a lovely way to celebrate Christmas."

Millie refused to budge. "No," she muttered, "But I'll have one on my birthday."

"Oh, that's a good idea." said Matron. "And when is your birthday?"

"Next May," growled Millie.


Minden said she was attending a patient when she heard a call from the end of the ward. "Nurse, nurse," said the voice, "come quickly, Walter has been bent over his chair for ages and hasn't said a word."

"I went quickly down the ward and bent over him. "What's wrong Walter?"

He lifted his head. "I'm trying to tie my shoelaces."

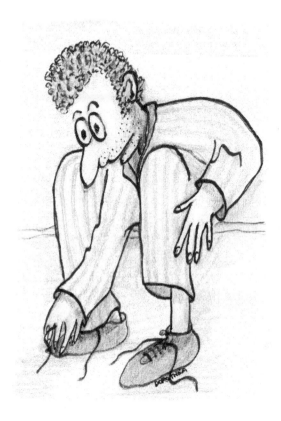

# OCCUPATIONAL THERAPY

Karen Bayston, Head Occupational Therapist, couldn't help but laugh when an elderly patient rang her to say she was having great difficulty with the wrist splints she'd been issued with. When she came into the department to show Karen the problem, she found she was putting them on inside out and upside down. "No wonder they didn't work." said Karen.

# ODD-BODS

Take George in the bed next to me, a small diffident man with the appearance of an undernourished clergyman. The first ten minutes of his morning ritual would begin with him blowing his nose. I swear his brains must be loosened with the force of the blasts - even worse, he looked in the tissue every time! - He then would trot off to the bathroom and do whatever men do in bathrooms, returning to finish his ablutions sat on his bed. First, after-shave would be liberally splashed over his face, followed by a deep massage of his cheeks. Deodorant was thrown with great abandonment under his arms, then he would tend to his toes. It looked like an atomic explosion the amount of talcum which surrounded his bed. The curtains would be drawn while he changed his pyjamas, carefully selecting a pair from the stockpile in his locker. My favourite was a red silk outfit with a mandarin collar and fetching gold tassels. He even had a perky little matching hat.

Further down the ward was probably the weirdest man I've ever come across Two tufts of orange hair, edged his pink scrubbed scalp. Although his frame was moderate he possessed the largest hands I've ever seen in my life. They looked like elephants ears. He would have made a wonderful subject for the wild-life artist David Shepherd! Every morning he asked for cornflakes, then mashed them up and walloped great spoons of marmalade on the top. He would then sit there, pale and red-eyed. blinking bleakly over the revolting mish-mash of breakfast.

I only ever saw him take two spoonfuls.

His wife was a large dominant person who constantly wore the same purple and pink floral dress. As soon as she sat down the questions began: "Have you washed your neck? Have you changed your pyjamas? Have you been to the lavatory to do your propers?

As Eve in the next bed remarked: "What's the point of having hands that big if you don't use them to wallop a few people."

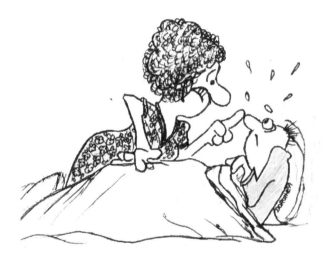

In the bed immediately opposite was Hilda who was constantly complaining. The nurses were puzzled as all her results had come back negative but her temperature kept leaping up and down like a yo-yo. It was in the days of mercury thermometers and the nurses would pop it into your mouth and leave you to 'cook' while administering the same to all the other patients. As soon as the nurse went on her way, she would either pop the thermometer into her water jug, which often had ice floating in the top, or into her hot cup of tea. As soon as the nurse turned round she would whip it out and place it back into her mouth. I'm afraid I spragged her, so they stood by her bed until the time was up - and her time definitely was.

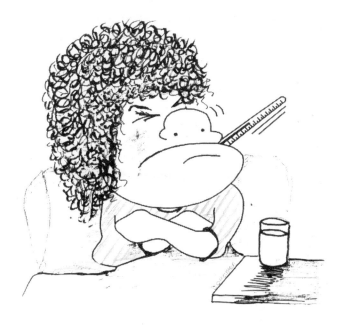

Later that day I watched in horror as the lady in the next bed intermittently spat into small pieces of torn newspaper. She would then give the top a neat little twist and the small parcel would be placed in a neat row on her bedside cabinet.

A nurse approached her bed. "Alice, what are you doing?"

"You said I had to keep my phlegm, so there it is."

"But I gave you a receptacle to put it in."

"Oh, I know, but it seemed a shame to dirty it."

After the nurse had gone, Alice leant over conspiratorially over to me. "Did you know you should always check your phlegm." she asked

"No," I said, "I didn't."

"Oh, yes." said Alice. "Very important. If it's white it's okay, but if it's yellow and smells of old socks it's ready to be coughed up. A bit like fruit really."

I daren't ask what she meant.

I was bed-bound and so was delighted when I found the next occupant to be my neighbour, was a real charmer. She lived in a world I had never frequented so listened with delight when she told me about her day to day happenings. She talked non-stop, all conversation littered with swear words. Boring she certainly wasn't.

"Have you got a dish-washer?" she asked.

"I do," I told her, "but I never use it."

"So do your kids do it?"

"I've only one and I don't know if he'd know where to start."

"Well I told me 'usband I wanted a bloody dish-washer so what did 'e bloody do? Only went out and bought me a fifty pence dish mop! So I told my lot they'd 'ave to do turns in doing the pots, our Jason didn't do bad or our 'chelle, but bloody Dave was something else. I couldn't understand why we kept needing new pots, even the knives and forks seemed to be disappearing, then one day I was taking out the rubbish, when I bloody 'eard rattling. I opened up the plastic bag and it was only bloody full of pots'n stuff. Our Dave 'ad been slinging 'em rather than wash 'em up. I soon sorted that. I kept one of everything just for mesen and let the others manage as best they could. They only used their bloody fingers, so I changed my cooking habits. I gave them stew, rice pudding, peas, mash, anything that caused a mess. The buggers only licked their bloody plates. I went ballistic, so me 'usband, Jeff went to an auction and bought two bags full of plastic plates and cutlery. They were from a cafe who'd gone bust. Mind you, it did solve the problem, everything was thrown out. Bloody made my life a lot easier I can tell you."

There were lots of other fascinating snippets of her home life but that was my favourite by far.

Charles was in a four bed ward in Castle Hill Hospital. The man next to him had hardly moved for three days. "I thought he must be dying," said Charles. "I had a young man opposite who was constantly complaining, usually about nothing in particular. One afternoon, I heard the young man say. "When I lie down, it really hurts'. Suddenly the comatose man next to me leapt upward and shouted. 'Well bloody well sit up then.' and returned to his comotose position."

Any new patients who had been settled in were all approached by Harry. He would stand by their bed, nod and with a broad grin announce; "I'd like to tell you a joke. It's not mucky." and without waiting would plough on regardless, "There was this man see who was looking 'round an antique shop and he spotted a mirror he particularly liked. The shop keeper said it was a magic mirror and would enlarge anything you placed in front of it. So the man bought it immediately, took it home and stood it against a wall. He stood in front of it, stark naked and said, 'mirror, mirror, can you make me one that touches the floor', in seconds his wish was obeyed. His legs fell off!" He would roar with laughter, exclaiming, "That's a good one yeah?"

Thank you Harry, but after the seventh time of telling, I found great difficulty in getting my smiley bits to work.

Gladys Whitaker said her sister-in-law Joyce can't stand the sound of snoring, so when in hospital she always puts on eye-shades and puts in ear plugs before settling down. "But one night," said Gladys, "a male patient was having a nightmare and leapt out screaming, this in turn woke up other male patients who thought a madman was on the loose and anyone capable of moving did so at great speed. The rest just lay there and yelled. Two managed to get into the female ward before nurses calmed things down and re-assured everyone. The next morning of course it was the talk of the ward, well to everyone except my sister-in-law, who's slept blissfully through the lot. But it gets better," she said.

"The following day, Joyce had her early morning cup of tea and the auxiliary was checking blood pressures and temperatures. The thermometer was one of those hand held ear probes The nurse popped it into Joyce's ear but couldn't get a reading. She changed it for another. Still no reading. Joyce suddenly realised. She hadn't taken out her earplugs!"

A nurse came to tell Doris that a man called Lenny would like to talk to her.

"Tell him I'm out."

"But he obviously knows you're here."

"I don't want to talk to him."

"Ever?"

"Ever!"

The nurse went to relay the message to Lenny, She returned to Doris.

"I told him, but I don't think I'll tell you what he told me to do."

"No, but I can bloody guess," said Doris.

It turned out he had a police order out not to molest her, but he was not easily deterred. He rang the hospital switchboard and hurled abuse at them, so the hospital contacted Kingston Communications to block the calls. They knew all about him. The police were informed and they came to interview Doris.

"Wow,!" said one of the nurses, "We haven't had so much excitement since one of the consultants ran off with a junior nurse."

I tried to glean more but her lips were firmly sealed.

An overweight female patient stopped by my bed to tell me: "I always get weighed after I've been to the lav. If I've got constipation I don't get weighed, 'cos I know the extra weight will only be shit! The bloody doctors are always telling me to lose weight, but I'm only sixteen bloody stone and I'm five-foot four. It's in your genes. I know somebody who died of a heart attack while he was bloody exercising, so I don't give a sod. But I bloody 'ate my sister-in-law. She's always telling me about bloody cholesterol and if I have salt, I'll snuff it. I'll lay you a penny to a fiver that she'll bloody snuff it before I do. Anyway I'm a lot 'appier than that miserable cow."

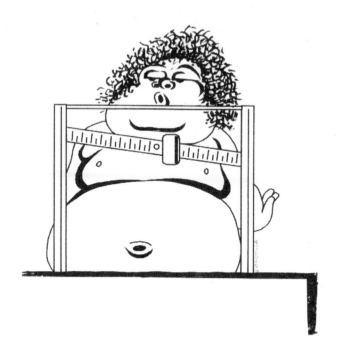

After imparting this scintillating piece of information she trolled back to her bed. She was discharged two days later but I was sorry to see this larger than life personality disappear, because I now realise I've led a pretty sheltered upbringing. Eccentric characters like her are not exactly ten-a-penny, but I'm glad I was able to have my two-pennyworth in what I now realise is a very cloistered life.

# OPERATIONS

I once saw an advertisement in a New Zealand newspaper:

"For sale: Surgical instruments. Complete assortment of deceased surgeons."

Up to now I have spent a total of two years in and out of hospitals, so when I was admitted to Castle Hill for a hip replacement, I thought I'd be a patient for 14/15 days but a few blood clots decided to have a wander around my anatomy admiring the scenery, eventually settling beautifully in my lungs and so extending my stay.

But first let me tell you about my comical operation.

I can't say it got off to the best start in the world. On the day before the operation, the surgeon, who I knew quite well, came to see me. He was having a lot of personal problems and decided to open his heart to me. Luckily I was in a single room, so he was able to chat freely for over half-an-hour. The bizarre events that had happened over the last three months had turned a handsome, articulate, talented man into almost giving up his profession.

Everybody assumed he had it all, a beautiful wife, happy, well adjusted children and a reputation second to none as a surgeon. But nothing could be further from the truth. I won't go into details, but suffice to say it nearly destroyed him. He now had no wife, no home, no children and no money. At the end of his tale of woe, I could only put my arms around him and give him a great hug.

"Do you know Dorothea," he said, "At the moment I hate coming into work in the mornings."

"Hey!" I said, slightly alarmed, "I'm on your list tomorrow."

"Oh, don't worry, I promise I'll be bright eyed and bushy tailed."

"Just bright eyed would be fine." He gave a wan smile. "Another promise," he said. "I will get through this. I have to haven't I?"

He left to start his ward rounds.

The following morning, I was woken at six am to have a bath.

"Why?" I asked, "The op's not until eleven."

"Oh, the surgeon has changed the rota and he's put you in first."

Well at least I could check if he was bright eyed and bushy tailed. I was wheeled to theatre for eight-thirty. This was familiar territory as four years previously I'd had my first hip replacement and had opted for an epidural. This is an injection in your spine, which deadens - you hope - the bottom half of your body but leaves the top half fully awake and aware of what's going on around you. On the first operation I'd been given a headset to listen to a musical tape, but the volume could not be turned up to obliterate the sounds I was keen to ignore, so this time my son had promised to prepare a tape that would definitely drown out the hub-bub of the theatre.

The day before surgery, Adam had presented me with a compilation of songs by Queen. I couldn't argue with his choice. They are loud!

Picture the scene: A trolley, complete with prone female being wheeled into an operating theatre with a tape of Queen nestling on her tum.

The anaesthetist, perched on a small chromium stool, took the tape, commenting, he liked Queen as he inserted the tape and popped the earphones onto his head to have a quick listen. I suddenly remembered the last op. where the anaesthetist was reading the morning paper, I could quite clearly hear the pages being turned and we also had some interesting conversations about the political content.

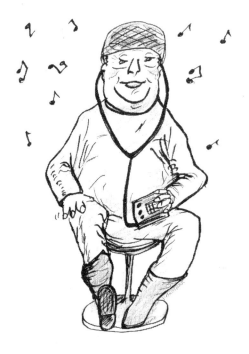

The operating table sat in the centre of a bare, tidy room, with large arc lamps suspended from the ceiling. The team consisted of the surgeon - and yes he was bright eyed and bushy tailed - the registrar surgeon, theatre sister, the anaesthetist, and I think two others, but who was counting, certainly not me! Concentration was not my strong point at this moment in time!. The thing that instantly struck me was the temperature, it was freezing. 'My God,' I thought, I hope they're all wearing thermals or they'll be shivering and shaking under their gowns and this was not an option I favoured, especially while wielding a sharp knife!

This time I was not aware of any leafing through pages of newsprint, but we had a fairly meaningful conversation about the merits of Kevin Keegan as England manager and Tony Blair's latest exploits. During a short pause I heard the surgeon call for a "six-inch saw". Queen were really strutting their stuff but I'm afraid it didn't even begin to drown out the hee-hawing of the saw.

Then I heard a crisp, "Mallet." The sound was horrific. There was nothing on God's earth which could persuade me they were not demolishing the theatre brick by brick. My eyes must have looked like chapel hat pegs. I steeled myself - well my top half anyway - I concentrated very hard on the music. I suddenly became aware of the words, I concentrated even harder, but no I hadn't misheard, I found the vocal histrionics of Freddie Mercury being used to belt out a song which had been lovingly selected by my son - I was being serenaded with 'Tie Your Mother Down'. I burst out laughing and held out the earphones for all to hear. I think we scored a first. Uncontrolled laughter in an operating theatre. The surgeon popped his head over the screen. "I must say I'm impressed by your son's sense of humour" he said, and went back to his chip, chip, chipping. We had another conversation about formula one racing, then I heard "more cement please." Was I really in an operating theatre or in a dream and had wandered into a building site. Suddenly the surgeon was by my side.

"All done Dorothea, it went really well. I haven't had such a laugh for ages." He gave me a knowing look as he squeezed my hand before returning to the theatre.

After a spell in the recovery room I was wheeled back to the ward, complete with oxygen mask, saline drip, blood bag and drains. Waiting for me were my husband and recalcitrant son.

He gave me a cheeky grin.

"I forgive you," I said and went on to say how it cheered not just me but all the theatre team.

He told me he'd thought about it carefully but decided as my sense of humour was as wacky as his, he would pop it in the middle of the tape.

Without doubt it had considerably lightened three turbulent hours.

Oh, I've just remembered another first. Just before the screens were placed in front of me, I could see a bright orange leg sticking straight up in the air. "Good grief," I thought, I couldn't even do that when I was fifteen! but I found out later it was because they have to dislocate it first before they start the operation. Uugghh!!

I was so impressed by my son's attempts to cheer me up I sent all my friends a poem about it.

Tales of mayhem, tales of woes,
Tales I promise will curl your toes.
I first gave the sexy doc. a cuddle,
Because his life was in such a muddle.

The theatre I was soon inside,
Now there was no-where I could hide,
The nurses then put up the screen
Their work should definitely not be seen.

Saws and chisels and cement called for,
"Please," I shouted, "Show me the door."
"You can't leave now," the doc replied,
"We need to open up your side."

Talk was on a higher plain,
I must admit I felt no pain,
Conversation soon changed tack,
Should they have taken Keegan back?

A group was playing in my ear,
And dear friends what did I hear?

142

My son's selection, he'd been very keen,
It was, "Tie Your Mother Down," by Queen.

The theatre staff were quite amused
and my son Adam verily accused,
of a sense of humour, quite bizarre,
but deeply appreciated by his Ma.

While being wheeled back to my room Hannah was heading towards the theatre. She waved and said: "Well done, it's me next."

She looked decidedly perky. "You look very relaxed," I called out to her.

"Relaxed! I'm about as relaxed as a turkey sat on a box of Paxo." she called out as the trolley disappeared down the corridor

As I mentioned I'd had an epidural for the operation and a morphine drip inserted in my back to assist with pain relief. This is a great improvement, as usually nurses have to pop in on a regular basis to administer injections, but this releases medication every twenty minutes or so, plus you have a button you can press if you feel you need a top up.

I was waxing lyrical to Molly about the advancement in surgical procedures. She gave me a knowing look, "Yes," she said, "I had one of those but a few hours after the op. I started to feel pain which increased considerably by the minute. Nurses came to investigate but decided all was well and gave me some oral pain killers. Eventually I was screaming at them to do something. It was midnight but they summoned a doctor immediately. He checked me thoroughly then discovered the morphine drip had been attached to the wrong hip. It was taken out but could not be put back so I was on the dreaded injections. It all turned out well in the end," said Molly, "But I was not a happy bunny for a few hours."

That must be the understatement of the year!

Jane, who was just recovering from a hand operation, said she wished she could have something you just pressed. At that moment a nurse walked by and she complained bitterly to her that the wound was quite painful.

"Don't worry," said Mandy, "Everything's fine. It's just knitting together."

"Is it now," said Jane. "Well I wish it would follow a plain pattern and not a complicated cable stitch."

Two days after my op. a lady opposite was being prepared for her hip replacement. I heard her ask the nurse: "Do I have to take my teeth out?"

"Are you having an epidural?" the nurse asked.

"No way. I don't want to hear what's going on. I want to be put to sleep."

"Well in that case you'll have to take your teeth out."

"Do I for both?"

"No, only the full anaesthetic."

"In that case I'll have the other thing and bung me ears up, 'cos nobodies seeing me with me teeth out."

# OUT-PATIENTS

While attending the out-patient department of Hull Royal Infirmary, I noticed this sign pinned to the wall behind the admissions clerk:
All targets met
All systems fully operational,
All customers satisfied,
All staff keen and motivated,
All pigs fed and ready to fly.

Wendy an auxiliary in the Accident & Emergency department, told me about a young fourteen year old who was having problems with spots.

"The clinic had suggested a specially formulated face wash for him. After about a month his mother brought him back, as they were not improving. They suggested he try another type of face wash. Still no improvement. Then one day his mother caught him going through his daily skin care routine before going out. Mum told the doc. that he was patting the individual spots with a blob of the wash and just leaving it. 'It's my fault,' said the mum, "I should have explained it."

A round rosy cheeked woman came to sit beside me. I noticed her leg was heavily bandaged, so asked what had happened.

"Well, I'd been feeding some wild cats at the back of my

garden, they've been there over a year. One was quite friendly and I put a line across the end of the garden with some toys hanging from it, so he could play. A couple of days ago I saw him sat in a bed of Petunias, so went out with some food for him, when I was a couple of feet away he suddenly pounced and clamped his jaws around my leg. He'd opened his mouth so wide he couldn't get free and his teeth were embedded in my leg. I was screaming and trying to shake him off, then my husband rushed out and started kicking it. It seemed ages before it eventually let go. Next door had heard the commotion and sent for an ambulance. When they came they couldn't stem the blood and when the doctor saw it he said they couldn't stitch it as it would cause problems, so I had to stay in hospital for a few days, but I'm not here with my leg. I'm here to check if I'm diabetic. Somebody once told me animals can be diabetic. You don't think I caught it from them mangy tom do you?" Before I could comment my name was called out and my consultant beckoned.

Margaret P. was asked to attend the out-patients department for an X-ray.

Her name was called and she entered the room. An African doctor asked her to 'take her knickers off.'

"I duly stepped out of my pale pink M & S briefs," said Margaret, "Only to my horror, I found out he was telling me to 'take my necklace off."

"As it was only the thorax, I should have realised, but I was brought up to 'always do as you are told."

Mrs Crow was waiting for her appointment with the consultant. She's been asked to bring a sample of her urine, which she'd put in a polystyrene cup. She placed it on the floor while she was waiting but accidentally kicked it over. A WRVS lady was just passing with her trolley and went to pick it up for her. "Shall I fill it up for you?" she asked, thinking she'd spilt her cup of tea.

# OVERHEARD

I was laid in bed ear-wigging any passing conversation, when I heard a patient say to a nurse: "I can't understand a word you're saying, don't forget I've got Liverpool ears. I haven't been 'ere long enough to get 'ull ears."

"How long have you lived here then?"

"Seventeen years."

"Bloody 'ell, you could 'ave grown elephants ears in that time."

A male nurse at Castle Hill had the wonderful name of James Cagney. He had previously been in the army and had a ready wit, usually at the patients expense. He was guaranteed to brighten a ward within minutes. No-one took offence and everyone looked forward to his cheery face when he came on duty.

An 84 year old had a very high temperature and after removing the thermometer, he checked it and with a cheeky grin, winked and said: "Wow, Mavis, I knew you were a bit of hot stuff. Do you think you could give my wife lessons?" Instead of being worried she gave him a great beaming smile.

Ada had been coughing for some time, when Jim suddenly appeared in the doorway and shouted: "Look, I'm trying to work in here so whoever's choking to death can they please do it quietly."

"What shall I do with these?" asked Maureen, holding up a pair of elastic stockings.

"I could think of somewhere you could stick 'em, but I don't think you'd like it." said Jim.

He was filling up everyone's water jugs with fresh water and ice cubes.

"Jim," called out Sheila, " My ice has melted."

"Bloody 'ell," said Jim, "The polar ice cap's melting and you're moaning about your ice cubes. I bet you'd moan if the queen came to tea 'cos it was your night at the bingo."

Teresa asked him if he was lucky.

"Me, lucky! You've got to be joking. I'm married aren't I? I tell you I'm so unlucky, that if I wanted to end it all and jumped off the Humber Bridge, the tide would be out and I'd plop into a nice soft mud bank."

While helping Sister on the drug round the banter still didn't stop. He informed the patients: "Watch out for that Cathy. She's got a mind of her own she has."

Suddenly a voice piped up: "Go on Jim tell me, who else's would she bloody 'ave?"

Jim was settling the patients down for the night, but Martha was not a happy bunny.

"I need to be higher," she told him.

"If I lift you any higher," said Jim, "You'll be in flaming heaven."

At the end of the evening while doling out the bedtime drinks he told the patients, "After looking after you women all day, I go home to my wife and give her a great big hug and a big passionate kiss."

"Why, do we all get you going?" asked Dorothy.

"No quite the opposite. I'm glad to be able to talk to someone normal for a change."

A small girl was waiting with her parents outside the children's ward, when a nurse came by pushing a stretcher. They paused for a moment and the patient asked the youngster if she was coming into the hospital.

"Oh, no," said the child. "I'm coming to see my brother."

"Oh, dear, I hope he's getting better," said the man.

"Oh, yes, he's eating ice-cream 'cos he's had his plimsolls out."

Visitor to patient. "What's the lav. paper like in here, is it the 'ard stuff?"

Patient to visitor. "Naw, it's the soft stuff, trouble is its only three inches wide. No bloody good to anybody. I use the morning paper."

Overheard: "My sister 'ad that done and she cut everything with one arm."

I don't think that will take over from a knife!

Now are you concentrating? Then I'll begin. First picture two beds side by side, in one sits tall, bony Bernice, about 60 with dyed black hair, tied back with a bright yellow spotted scarf, in the second bed sits Pauline, early 40's orange, permed hair and wearing a green and purple striped nightie. Bernice lifts up her water glass.

"You see that? I've got a mucky glass and I'm not allowed to complain. I 'ate it, I really 'ate it, but I always get chowed at if I complain."

"Do you want mine?"

"No I bloody don't." And without drawing breath. "Where do you 'ave your 'air cut?"

"Bernard's opposite the Criterion."

"Oh, yes, my mate always goes there but he died last year"

"He didn't 'cos I went there last week and saw him."

"He did 'cos he was my mate."

"Bernard?"

"No, my mate."

"Is 'e dead then?"

"Who?"

"Whoever you're talking about."

"Bernard or me friend."

"Either. Is 'e dead?"

"I don't think so."

And with that swung her marbled limbs out of bed and toddled off to the loo.

Brenda was the mandatory complaining patient. She invariably found something to moan about. Nurses usually gave her a wide berth, unless it was absolutely essential.

So there we were being woken at 6.30am by the tea trolley rattling its way up the ward.

"All right everybody?" enquired the nurse as she doled out the cheering cuppa.

"No, I'm not all right," moaned Brenda. "I never slept a wink. I couldn't get my legs comfortable all night."

"Oh, what a shame," said the nurse. "You should have tried wrapping them around your neck, that would have done the trick."

Couldn't have put it better myself.

Ward seventy had more than its share of eccentric patients. One day during visiting Muriel had three friends sat at her bedside. I heard one comment: "I hope you don't mind me not sending you a card, but I never buy one if it's over fifty pence."

"Don't worry," said her friend, "I don't expect a card."

One of her other visitors chipped in. "What she didn't tell you was, we all went to get you a card and she could have had one for fifty-one pence, but she wouldn't buy it. We both offered her the extra penny, but she wouldn't budge."

"Principles is principles and fifty one pence is more than fifty pence. You understand don't you Muriel?"

Muriel nodded dumbly.

The lady in the next bed was recovering from a bladder operation, but she was having a slight problem. She couldn't' stop dribbling. Two very elegant ladies came to visit her in the afternoon and she was explaining her dilemma to these apparently cultured women. I heard one say loudly: "Oh, dear how awful Veronica, you can never feel really smart with wet knickers can you?"

"Why hasn't our Hilda come to see me?"
"Her chest is bad."
"Oh. What's wrong then?"
"Just 'er chest."
"What brought that on then?"
"She said she went into the garden with her slippers on."
"That'd do it."

Mrs Watson confided in a nurse that she was worried what her husband was getting up to while she was in hospital.
"Why, what do you think he might be up to?" asked the nurse.
"Well, the last time I was in here for ten days and you should have seen the mess when I got home. Pots and pans were piled high in the sink and you couldn't see the draining board. Do you know?" she whispered, "He'd even been upstairs into the loft and brought out the old wicker picnic basket and used all the plastic plates."
"Is that all? I thought you meant hanky-panky."
"Hanky-panky! Good God" exclaimed the patient. "The only hankie pankie he knows about is the one you blow your nose on."

There was a general conversation going on about a variety of subjects when a patient asked: "What's that you pick up in swimming baths? You know you get it on your feet."
Another lady called out. "That's a verouk. isn't it?"
"Naw." said Julie, "He was an Egyptian King wasn't he?"

Nurse: "Sit back Edith."

Patient: "I can't sit back any further, my legs are too long."

Nurse: "Rubbish. Do what I did."

Patient: "What's that then?"

Nurse: "Run around the ward and wear them down. I used to be 5'8 you know. I'm only 5'5 now."

Patient: "Don't be silly."

Nurse: "Silly? Look at me Edith. Do I look more than 5'5?"

Patient: "No. I know you're not."

Nurse: "There you are then."

Sister Smith, overheard the following conversation between a volunteer, who was changing flowers in the ward and a very morose patient.

"What are you in for?"

"No idea. I couldn't breathe so they rushed me in."

"Oh, dear," said the flower lady," don't worry, it's not so bad, I've been in three times."

The patient didn't answer.

"Yes and all with the same thing." The patient still ignored her. But the voluntary worker persevered. "I've had three hip replacements."

"She obviously thought that would impress the patient," said Sister Smith, "But no response, so she announced what she thought was her coup de` Gras".

"One's been done twice!"

The patient looked disparagingly at the flower lady and muttered.

"Yes, well I didn't think you 'ad three legs, anyway, everyone's ill when there's summat wrong wi` 'em. Stands to reason."

As Sister Smith commented, "I couldn't argue with that."

Claire had asked for a bedpan and Janet, the auxiliary, duly took one to her. She drew the curtains and I overheard Janet telling Claire to: "Shove your finger on that little hole, then it wont run so fast."

There was no answer from the patient. The nurse reappeared leaving the curtains drawn and busied herself about the ward.

I called her over. "Now I know it's not really any of my business, but what on earth were you talking about to Claire?"

"Oh she was trying to drink one of those cartons of blackcurrant and it was coming too fast up the straw."

Cor. What a relief!


Overheard in the surgical ward.

"We play dominoes every Tuesday, but missed yesterday 'cos I was in 'ere. It was the bloody final as well."

The lady in the adjacent bed asked her. "Was there any prizes?"

"Bloody was. The winners got a bottle of whisky and second, some wine."

"No, I mean proper prizes."

"What do you mean proper prizes." Righteous indignation flared from her eyes. "They are proper prizes."

"No they're not, money's a proper prize."

"What a load of bullshit. You've obviously never won anything in your life."

And with that turned away, a very miffed lady.


On the twelfth floor of Hull Royal Infirmary, you can see the River Humber and a bed near the window can be quite relaxing - on a clear day you understand - Anyway Dora was contentedly gazing out, well as contented as you can be with both ends severely bunged up! I wont go into details! Suddenly she screamed and two nurses came running. "Whatever's the matter Dora?"

"I just saw an enormous piece of masonry fall from the roof. The building's crumbling. Somebody ought to check straight away."

A lady in the bed opposite, who had also been Humber gazing, butted in. "Sorry, nurse, but I saw it as well. It was only a pigeon swooping down."

Dora was not convinced and asked to be moved nearer the centre of the ward.

It was early morning and the ward was being woken from their slumbers. The patients bed opposite me was a real mess.

"Blimey," she said, "Did I have a fellah in here last night?"

"From the look of your bed," replied the nurse, "More like ten fellahs."

"Oh dear God. I must have slept through the whole thing. Tell me Sheila, did I enjoy it."

With a twinkle in her eye the nurse said,. "Couldn't tell you, but I notice your purse is full."

A patient was lying quietly in bed reading a magazine, when a young nurse approached. "Come on Maisie, up you get. We need to change your bed."

A large smile enveloped the patients face and as the nurse disappeared through a door she climbed out of her bed and went to inspect a spare one at the end of the ward, sat on it, then started to move her things across the room. The nurse returned. "What are you doing?" she asked.

"You said change beds."

The nurse had to explain that it was only the bedclothes that were being changed.

Honor was telling us about her daughter.

"I paid for over eighty driving lessons for her. It was an old chap what took 'er and 'e said she wasn't ready. When will she be bloody ready I asked. She was convinced she was ready. I told her to ignore the silly old sod and put in for it, so she did, but it was another old bloke that took her for the test. He only went and bloody failed 'er, so she's given it up, mind you," she said, wagging her finger at me. "It 'asn't stopped 'er. She always drives when they take the kids out."

It was early morning and I'd got up to go to the loo, as I passed a bed, the occupant asked "What time is it?"

"Quarter past five," I whispered and carried on. She then started talking to the patient next to her - very loudly - A nurse came and asked her to "Keep it down, please, most of the patients are still asleep."

"Keep it down! I will not keep it down. After all I've had to put up with all night. Tell that noisy bugger over there to keep it down. There she is snoring away and she kept me awake all bloody night."

"She wasn't very well." said the nurse timidly.

"Yes, well I'm not very well, so let's see how she likes it." and continued shouting loudly to a nearby patient who was hiding her head under the bedclothes. It didn't make a scrap of difference and she carried on. The nurse was only young and was not sure how to handle the cantankerous old woman, so discreetly tip-toed out.

During the night a nurse had to attend to Maria on several occasions. She was still awake at 3.30am so the nurse asked if she'd like a cup of tea. "I'd love one," said Maria. "No sugar." The nurse went. At 6.30am the ward was being woken and the nurse went over to Maria. "I did bring you that cup of tea but you'd already fallen asleep."

"I didn't fall asleep for ages," said Maria, "I was waiting for you."

"Oh well," said the nurse, "it was probably an hour or so before I did find time to bring it. Shame you'd nodded off though, you would have enjoyed it."

Maria was speechless.

Betty was being visited by her son-in-law. You know the type, blonde streaks, designer labels and the ubiquitous mobile hung from his belt. "When might you be out then?" he asked.

"Well they say it could be tomorrow, but only if I've got transport."

"Transport? What are they talking about? There's a bus stop outside the bloody hospital."

Betty was 72, arthritic and walked with two sticks. And no, he wasn't joking!

Cathy the staff nurse was never at a loss for the ready quip and put down. Sample:

Patient: What are these pills?"
Cathy: Don't ask me. I don't know.
Patient: Well you gave 'em to me."
Cathy: You've been taking them long enough.
Patient: Yes, but there's a yellow one, I haven't seen before.
Cathy: Oh, don't worry about it. That's arsenic.
Patient: Are you trying to polish me off?"
Cathy: Don't tempt me Mildred, don't tempt me.

On the same medicine round a patient suddenly appeared fully dressed, with a hold-all hanging over her shoulder. At that moment Cathy was giving an injection to a patient so didn't see her. The figure headed for the outside door - we were in a single story building where the wards overlooked lawns - the woman was muttering: "I've been insulted and they've been messing with my bed. They needn't think they can talk to me like that. Insulting that's what it is." In a split second the door was open and she was gone. We all shouted to Cathy: "Oh God I know who that'll be," she said and quickly locking the drugs cabinet, took off after her. She returned only moments later holding aloft the hold-all. "Don't worry," she said, "She'll not go far without this." She put it on a nearby chair and carried on as if nothing had happened. She was right, after her bag had been purloined, the patient made herself comfortable in a plastic garden chair and it was two hours before she agreed to return.

Patient: Are these pain killers?"

Cathy: Ah, that's where you have to trust me.

Patient: I'm only asking.

Cathy: Well I'm not telling.

Cathy returned after placing a thermometer under the Josie's arm.

"Are you cooked yet?"

"It hasn't bleeped yet," replied Josie.

"You mean you never knew the magic moment when you bleeped?"

"No I never heard a thing."

"God, just think, it's like sex, you could have laid back and thought of England, while you enjoyed your very own bleep."

"I never enjoyed sex, so I'm damn sure I wasn't going to think of England while a thermometer bleeped under my smelly armpit."

Ah, well, you can't win 'em all Cathy.


"Can I have two pain-killers?"

"Strong or medium?" asked Cathy.

"What's the difference?"

"That's a bloody silly question. One's strong and one's not so strong."

"What do you think?"

"Don't ask me, I haven't got the pain."

"Yes, but what do you think is best?"

"I know," said Cathy, "Have one strong and one medium, that should do the trick"

"What if it doesn't?"

"I've got the perfect remedy."

"What's that then?"

"I hit you over the head with a hammer."


A new patient had been admitted late the previous evening

and she soon met the indomitable Cathy.

"Morning May. Night staff tell me you're a troublemaker."

May giggled.

"Never mind giggling. This is serious. For troublemakers I offer two choices. You can either have a laxative every three hours or five soap and water enemas."

Helen was proving difficult to put to bed.

"I prefer the wheelchair, it's really, really comfortable."

"We can soon sort that out:" said Staff Nurse Cathy, "We'll get it grafted to your bum."

"Do you have a problem with your bowels?" asked Cathy.

"I'll have to put my glasses on first." said Wilma

"I hardly dare ask," said Cathy, "But before you do what?"

The patient giggled. "Oh, not to go to the lav. just to see who I'm talking to."

"That's a relief," said Cathy

Sister came in smiling. "I've heard everything now." she told Cathy, "I've just had a man on the phone who asked me if the results for Mr Thomas were all clear. I asked him who was enquiring. Do you know what he said?"

Cathy shook her head.

"It's Mr Thomas. Nobody tells me anything in the ward, so I thought I'd try a different approach."

"I've come to take your clips out." said a nurse as she pulled the curtains around Shirley's bed.

I could hear every word.

"Ooohh, I've been dreading this." said the patient.

"Have you? Why?" asked the nurse.

"I just have. I hate anything like this."

"Why don't you watch what I'm doing, that might help."

"You've got to be joking. I'm not a looker."

"You can say that again." Luckily the inference was lost on this patient..

"No I couldn't even peep. Is anybody lookers?"

"Oh, we have a few, but not at the moment." There was a short pause. "Are you all right?"

Deep intake of breath. "Sort of." said the patient.

"Sort of." exclaimed a triumphant nurse. "I'm having a ball."

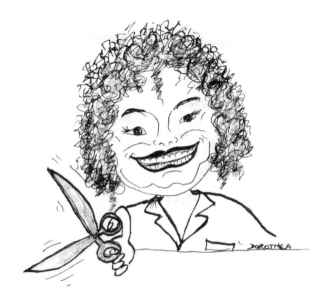

The cleaning staff were clearing tables of crockery and changing the jugs of water. I also had two very small pill containers on my table to take but she only cleared one away.

"You've left one," I called out helpfully.

She glared at me and muttered: "Do you realise I've got to wash those bloody things up."

# STUDENT NURSES

Nurses have a thorough training and have to sit many exams. A training sister - by the way her surname was Patient - told me: "They see a question staring them in the face but even though they know the answer, because they're under pressure, they become flustered and end up putting a very silly answer. A lot of students consider final examinations a bit like death. Inevitable, but you have to face them sooner or later."

"When I'm on duty during written exam's, there isn't a sound in the room while they are in progress and the nervous tension is palpable and there is a lot of pale faces as they file out to await their fate. But I think oral examinations are even more nerve wracking. It's probably something to do with the physical contact with examiners which make them so frightening. The written papers have a sort of remoteness about them, but in the oral exam when you suddenly realise you've made a monumental clanger, your mind goes blank as you're are faced with a row of expressionless faces. You're convinced it will be castration at least!"

She then revealed some of the clangers made by nervous students.

Q. How should you treat patients suffering from shock?
A. Rape them up in blankets.

Q. State the difference between psychiatrists and psychologists.
A. They're different in that they're the same.

Q. What is artificial respiration commonly known as?
A. The kiss of death.

Q. How can parents help when a child wakes in the night suffering from breathing difficulties?
A. Make them inhale a steam kettle.

Q. From what may men in their fifties suffer?
A. The manopause.

Q. What is the common treatment for a bleeding nose?
A. Circumcision.

Q. Why do prescription drugs vary from the over-the counter drugs?
A. Some drugs have a more lusting effect.

Q. People who suffer from insomnia are called what?
A. Insomniaphobics.

Q. What is a molar?
A. The small bone in your toe next to the big one.

Q. How must nurses prepare a patient before a pre-med injection?
A. They must wash a patients groin and genial areas.

Q. What do the letters NHS stand for?
A. Non Hospital Surgery.

Q. What are the major symptoms associated with VD?
A. Sufferers from VD may get an inflammable penis.

Q. If a person is feeling unwell, are they still allowed to be serving food?

A.  No, deceased people should not be allowed to serve food.

Q.  What is the function of antibodies?
A.  Antibodies are organisations in dispute with people.

And finishing with one told to me by a school teacher, but it has hospital connotations.

Q.  What may happen when a low front crosses a hilly area?
A.  It rains steroids.

In the 60's, while nurses were in training they stayed in a 'Home' attached to the Beverley Westwood Hospital. At this time it was very rare for men to take up this profession.

Allan Rowlands, a nurse, told me: "I was the only male among fifty females in the home and everyone was convinced I must be effeminate."

"The Sister and Clinical Assistant Matron had a separate sitting room. They owned a record player and I heard that sister had bought a record from the top twenty in the hit parade. I was very impressed. I just couldn't believe that this monster even knew about the top twenty!"

"We were woken every morning in time for work, but if it was our day off we were served breakfast in bed. We did have a dining room which was used by all staff, but any time matron, or in fact any senior staff member came into the room we had to immediately put down our knives and forks and stand to attention. Sometimes we were bobbing up and down the whole of our meal"

"Relatives were permitted to visit their offspring in the nurses home, but under no circumstances were children allowed inside and there was always a porter on duty to make sure no unwanted visitors slipped by. The nurses had to go outside to see their younger siblings and if it was raining the poor little things had to sit with the porter in his lodge."

"There was an 11.00 o'clock curfew and woe betide you if you were even a minute over. Twice a week we were allowed to stay out until 12.30. Nearly all the girls would go dancing at the Regal ballroom. One night the nurses were dancing away merrily when they suddenly realised they were going to miss curfew. Partners were left stranded in the middle of the floor. Coats were hurriedly retrieved from the cloakroom and the three raced back across the Westwood. They arrived breathless, but four minutes late. Muriel saw a sash window nearby which was open sufficiently for them to climb through. The lights were on and curtains drawn but they thought nothing of it. Janet went first. She climbed over the sill and disappeared into the room, followed by Muriel. Dorothy, after a furtive look round, clamped her hands on the sill and started to clamber in, as she pushed her head through the curtains she was aware of someone watching. She looked up. There was Sister glaring down at her, hands clasped behind her back and foot tapping furiously. They'd all climbed into her office in the middle of a meeting. They were grounded for a month."

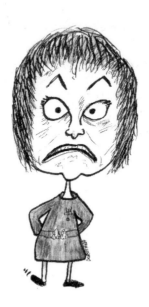

I asked Allan what the wages were like. "Very, very low," he told me. "In fact at the end of every month we were always completely skint. On the last week we would all sit round a table and pool our limited resources. Everybody smoked in those days, so we usually had just enough for ten Woodbines and a bottle of cider. As a cheap alternative we once tried a home brew cider kit. Trouble was it had to be left for a few days while it settled, but Andrea couldn't wait and sampled it before time. I can vouch it is not a sensible thing to do," said Allan, "She was really, really ill."

"If we didn't have enough for fags or cider we often went for a walk on the Westwood, but one night we decided it would be a good idea to sit under a tree and tell ghost stories, but with the full moon casting weird and wonderful shadows among the shrubbery, our imaginations started to run wild. We ended up running back to the nurses home in absolute terror, convinced something terrible was chasing us, especially a young girl from Barbados, whose surname was Nurse." He laughed. "None of us would believe it really was her surname. Everybody loved it, especially when Sister called out Nurse Nurse."

"One of our favourite haunts was Nellie Collinson's pub, the 'White Horse,' but known affectionately by everyone as 'Nellies.'"

"Nellie knew all the nurses and she always refused to serve any of the ladies with a pint glass and us males were never allowed more than two pints of Nellie's Old. 'We'll go somewhere else,' we told her, and her reply was always the same. 'Fair enough, off you go then, but I'll tell Sister.'"

"In all wards the matron reigned supreme and there was always a manic hustle and bustle to get the ward shipshape before she started her rounds."

"The preparation for her visit would start at six am! We had to scrub everything in sight, including the patients. Their lockers, always a jumble of drinks, flowers and newspapers, had to be stripped bare and the contents put out of sight. All beds had to be the same height and pillows had to have their open ends facing the main doors and the turn down flap of the sheet had to be 'fist

164

to elbow' length. On one ward the floor was tiled and she insisted all the beds were placed four and a half tiles apart. Not four and quarter or five but exactly four and a half, and you had to make sure all the beds wheels were pinchy toed - that's facing inward. Even patients were tidied, they were all told to get into bed. Sitting ON the bed was definitely taboo. We were told to pull the bedclothes really taut, which we did, but the poor patients were cocooned like a mummy and couldn't move anything. Just before the dreaded arrival all patients had to use a bedpan, whether they wanted to or not."

"What happened if she didn't think your handiwork was up to scratch?"

"Sometimes you got a rollicking on the spot, but it was not unusual for her to finish the round without a word. We would relax and give a sigh of relief and go for a tea break. But on our return we would find she'd stripped any offending beds and thrown the contents on the floor."

"Not including the patient I hope." He laughed. "No, but I think it was a near thing sometimes."

Margaret Whittaker was a student nurse at a psychiatric hospital. She told me:

"All the wards were called after females. I worked in Hannah and Naomi wards. There were some wonderful characters there, in fact I often joined them in their escapades. I often got asked when I was being discharged. This was because they thought I was one of them. We had one patient who had strangled three alsations, but we had to keep her in solitary in case she felt like trying it again on some of the old ladies paddling around. She was at least six feet tall and very athletic. She would perform the most amazing somersaults and cartwheels across the bedroom floor. It looked great fun and I would have loved to have joined her."

"Naomi Ward was the admission ward and I met a patient who had just been admitted because she'd tried to commit suicide by tying a pair of tights around the banisters then around her neck, except the tights stretched so much she plunged down to floor level and was unable to perform the dastardly deed. I asked her what sort of tights they were and she told me, 'Pretty Polly, so I told her she should write to the company telling them how wonderful the tights were. Tell them the elasticity saved your life."

"Did she?" I asked. "Dont think so." said Margaret.

Oh what a shame, I'd love to have known what the publicity boys had made of that.

"What sort of ages were the patients?" I asked

"Between 17 and 93," she said, "but most were elderly. We had one old dear who used to regularly go out for the day in a chauffeur driven Bentley. We had a fair few who wore hearing aids. Madge used to wear a striped one, which looked like a giant gob-stopper. When you took it out it was always sticky. I used to wonder if you could wash hearing aids.

"One day I noticed she wasn't wearing it, 'It's in the drawer' she told me, 'listening to everything you say'.

"When I left she said she had a present for me. I was delighted. Then I saw it and I wasn't so sure. She presented me with her hearing aid, sticky goo and all."

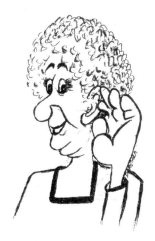

"Did you enjoy being there?" I asked.

"Oh loved every minute," she said, "but I had a lot of responsibility. During my time there I hardly ever saw the sister. She would ensconce herself in her room chain smoking and drinking herself into a mild stupor with gin. She would burn incense to try and cover the smell."

I loved talking to this charismatic seventy year old. She had some wonderful stories to tell of her schooldays in the 1930's. Must arrange to meet again.

Back on the hospital wards I heard a patient tell a nurse she was "bunged up."

"Don't worry, I'll get you something," said Nurse Walton.

As she was walking away the sister called for her urgently for some assistance in a side ward, so she told a student nurse to get something for Agnes. When she returned twenty minutes later, she saw the patient sat rigidly up in her bed with a suppository stuck up each nostril.

"They're not working." complained Agnes.

As nurse Walton said to me, "God knows where she puts her Vick's Nasal spray."

The pharmacist had just delivered the medication prescribed for patients who were being discharged. The staff nurse asked a student to take them round to the patients. "There were only two," said Maggie, "so I gave a packet of various pills and potions to a Mrs Black. The second was for a May Harmor. I checked the list but couldn't find a patient of that name. I went to ask Staff and she said we hadn't a Harmor on the ward and it had obviously been mis-delivered. I rang admissions and they couldn't find anyone with that name, so in desperation I rang the dispensary She was gone for ages then came back and said the medication was for Mrs Planter. Why doesn't it say that? I asked indignantly. We did, she told me, you were reading the instructions. I looked more closely. On the first line it read 'May harm or' and continued on the next line, 'discolour your urine."

A doctor in an East Yorkshire village was going out with a student nurse and he couldn't resist telling me about her first day in a ward. The senior nurses had shown her a bath thermometer, but told the hapless student it was really a rectal thermometer. She was despatched to take the temperature of a nearby patient .

Marie walked nervously to the bedside of Mr J., drawing the curtains she asked the patient to, "Lie on your stomach please." Just as she was about to insert this nine inch monstrosity in the rectum of the prostrate patient, the cavalry arrived, in the form of the staff nurse.

Student nurse Danielle said she thought she was being helpful when she filled a bowl beside a patients bed with warm water ready for her morning wash. Around the corner came a consultant on his rounds, so the senior nurse grabbed the bowl to secrete in the cupboard, not knowing it was full of water. The lot cascaded over the patient, floor, visiting consultant and entourage. He carried on, while nurses scurried around changing bed linen and poor Danielle was on her hands and knees spreading paper towels for the consultant to walk on.

Stories about teeth are rife in hospital and nearly all concern students. Moira told me: "I asked a junior nurse to clean several sets of teeth. She took them into the kitchen and emptied them into a bowl. Then of course no-one knew whose teeth belonged to which patient. We asked all the patients to try them. Most found a good home, except one elderly lady who pronounced that the ones in her mouth were definitely hers. We knew they couldn't be, `cos the top set were so big, they were on the outside of her lips. We all tried to persuade her to part with the teeth, but to no avail. She wouldn't even take them out when she snuggled down for the night. We waited `till she was sound asleep, then swopped them for the spare ones. She never complained so we`d got away with it."

Jane Woods told me about a student nurse who had been asked to "Take all the patients teeth into the kitchen and wash them." "She duly put them in the sink and scrubbed them thoroughly," said Jane, " thinking how pleased Sister would be with her efforts. They were then rinsed and put on the draining board. Then the awful truth dawned, she hadn't a clue which teeth went in which pot. There were five sets, some patients recognised their own, but it still left two sets. Sister told her that the patients would just have to try them out."

"Ron was the first to try out a set. 'These are fine,' he said: 'Definitely mine.'

"The other set were taken to Bernard. He put them in and immediately spit them out declaring. 'These aren't my bloody teeth."

"The young nurse protested that they were they were the only ones left,"

"I don't care, said Bernard, 'They're not mine."

The offending teeth were taken away and the nurse apprehensively approached Ron again. She explained the situation. Ron thought it a huge joke and relinquished the set he'd happily been chewing toffees on for the last five minutes. "Anything else you'd like me to test drive" he asked her."

"Bernard was not impressed with the proceedings and insisted the nurse scrubbed every morsel of toffee from them. When she returned, he tried them but and insisted he could still taste toffee. He sent the hapless girl back three times before he would wear them."

It was Boxing Day and the nurses were handing round sweets. Vera, a very vocal patient, shouted, "Where's mine then?" Janet went across and gave her one of those large toffee pennies. "'Bout time," said Vera, unwrapped it and popped it into her mouth. About half-an-hour had elapsed and nothing had been heard from Vera, so the young student went to see her. "She couldn't speak," said Janet, "the toffee had completely stuck her dentures together. It took two of us to release them."

In the olden days, probationers were called `Buttercups` and Minden recalled the time a `Buttercup` had been instructed to scrub the floor at a mental institution.

The probationer was down on her hands and knees, her pert bottom in the air, moving provocatively side to side as she scrubbed industriously. Sister came into the hall and was mortified to see a line of male patients with their trousers opened and obvious signs of great excitement, taking a great interest in the little `scrubber.`

A student who always had a happy smile and ready quip was checking if all the patients were comfortable.
"Everything okay?" she asked.
"Yes thank you Dooreen," said a strident voice nearby.
"Actually Gloria, it's pronounced Dureen."
"Oh pardon me, I'm sure," answered a very miffed patient. "You'll tell me next you went to university."
"I did actually," said Doreen.
"Bloody stuck up bitch."
The patient never spoke to her again.

Gill, a young nurse had been sent to administer a glycerine suppository to a patient.
"It was the first time I'd ever done it, so thought I'd better explain what I was going to do and quick as a flash the patient said to me, `don't put them in the wrong orifice will you, I don't want any jelly babies.`"

It was August and we were in the middle of a heatwave. A patient was constantly complaining.
Patient: "It's too hot in here. I can't stand it any more."
Sister: "It's hot for everybody. We're all hot."
Patient: "You can't be as hot as me. You've got to do something."
Sister by now was getting slightly irritated and called out.

"Nurse." A young student dutifully came over. "Yes, sister?"

Sister: "Go and get Nurse Thomas and then the two of you can push Mrs Carling's bed into the car park for the rest of the day."

I don't know whose face had the most interesting expression, the student nurse or the patient.

Cottingham hospital boasted a patient who had a glass eye. Sylvia told me:

"Last thing at night he would take it out, pop it in a saucer on the bedside table and first thing every morning, standing by his bed, he would take it and pop it back in its socket, he would then stride to some unsuspecting patient and looking them straight in the eye, would ask, `Is it in straight?`"

I know most of my anecdotes have been comic and I hope many made you smile but like everyone else I have had my dark and distressing times. Apprehension for painful and unpleasant treatment, which had to be endured with resignation. I was aching, sore, tender and unable to eat for weeks at a time. It was disagreeable and uncomfortable but I was always allowed my dignity. I never became complacent and however traumatic, I managed to sustain a sort of joie de vivre.

I never agonised over my illness or what the future held. I faced each day with an optimistic outlook and an eager expectancy. My restoration to health was never in question.

I am lucky to have a receptive disposition and a propensity for fun and I'm a complete romantic at heart. I never despaired - although I can't say the same for my family - I knew I would weather the storm.

But I did have one moment for which I was not so upbeat. It happened a week after I was discharged from my seven month stay in the infirmary. My face was swollen with cortisone. It was moon-faced and not the slender shape everyone remembered. My hair had lost its sheen and had turned a steely grey, hanging around my shoulders like an old lace curtain. My friends old me I looked fine and it wasn't nearly as bad as I thought. I tried very hard to ignore the image which stared back at me in the mirror. I had to believe them. They were adamant. One day there was a knock at the door, on the threshold stood an acquaintance I'd known quite well, two years earlier. She smiled and asked. "Is Dorothea in?"

Oh, dear, all my misgivings were now set in concrete.

There was another incident that I witnessed in 1999 that horrified me, and I'd like to share it with you. It was distressing, lamentable and extremely unpalatable and to be honest I can't conjure up a word which adequately describes my emotions at the time.

Let me set the scene. I was recovering after a hip replacement and the doctors suspected I may have blood clots, so I'd been sent, with another patient, to a hospital in Hull for a lung scan. After we had been 'scanned' we were taken to the ground floor to wait for an ambulance to return us to our host hospital. Eventually a paramedic approached us. "I can only take one at a time," he told the nurse accompanying us. "Which one is the most serious?" The nurse pointed to me. "Take the hip lady," he said, "the other is terminal."

I gasped and could only mutter, "We're all terminal. You included."

I found out later that my companion had been informed, only the previous day, that she only had a few months to live. The comment was inexcusable and that nurses insensitivity will haunt me forever.

Modern day nursing often leaves a lot to be desired, but while auxiliary's race around attending to patients needs, highly trained nurses and doctors are left to fill out forms.

I know hospital is not a fun place to be and most patients are apprehensive and anxious, but with a little foresight and planning it could be a damn sight more tolerable for everyone.

But let's finish with a smile.

A patient of the male gender was giving the nurses a bit of trouble. He refused to get into bed.

Sister was called for and she had a quiet word. All to no avail, so sister firmly told him to, "Get into bed this minute."

If she'd said it to me I'd have leapt in and cowered under the bedclothes for at least an hour.

But no, Arthur was having none of it. He replied. "I'll only get into bed if I can f*** that young blonde nurse."

Sister came over to the young auxiliary nurse standing near my bed and gently taking the girl by the arm said. "You'll have to do it Nurse Stathers, we can't sedate him at his age, and on this ward I'm afraid it's part of your duties."

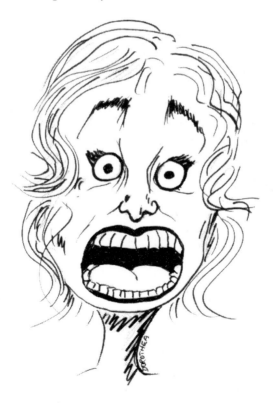

The nurse was speechless, not having worked on the ward for very long, or having met a sister with such a wicked sense of humour. She turned to me, mouth open and eyes wide with disbelief, but my face was wreathed in smiles, so she breathed a sigh of relief, turned and headed for Arthur. Sister and I watched as Joanne marched up to him and with hands on hips said: "Okay Arthur, I'm game if you are." Sister gave an audible gulp. "Oh, no," she gasped. "This is a dangerous game." But the come-uppance was absolute. Arthur's mouth opened even wider than the young nurse's and he turned niftily on his heels and climbed into bed, pulling the clothes over his head.

Sister was impressed "I wouldn't believe you could do it. That old fellah has more life in him than a tramps vest. I usually have to get doctor to sedate him." "Round one to us I think," said Sister.

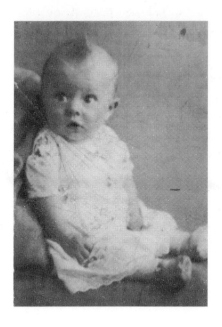

# About the author

Dorothea now lives in East Yorkshire with her husband Ray and two
Siamese cats. Her son Adam is an actor.

She has completed four other books – details overleaf.

Her next book 'Bands, Booze and Ballrooms'
is due out at Christmas 2001.
It's a nostalgic peep into the dance-band era,
full of anecdotes and photographs from 1940 to 1990.

# Other books:

### The Shocking Truth
Another humorous insight into the lives of Yorkshire folk, this time
through the eyes of a market researcher. (with illustrations)
Price £6.99

### Travel, The Celebrity Way
Anecdotes from 130 famous personalities, including, Rolf Harris,
Matthew Kelly, John Nettles, Richard Branson and John Prescott MP.
You're regaled with tales of hysterical honeymoons, cocky camels and
paralytic porters, with a sprinkling of murderous mountains, broken
bones and galloping goats.
Price £6.99

### The In-between Years 1940-1945
An evacuee's evocative account of her time in the Canadian
Prairies (with photographs)
Price £7.00

### Beyond the Brave
From Britain to bears, blizzards and buffalo.
A powerful portrayal of Canadian pioneers 1880-1946.
Price £7.99

All books can be obtained by writing to:
Buttercup Press, Ferry Road, South Cave,
East Yorkshire, HU15 2JG

Please add £1.20 for postage and packing (UK only).
Cheques to be made payable to T. James.